Intermittent Fasting For Women Over 50

Harness the Power of Time-Restricted Eating to Optimize Weight, Wellness, and Longevity

Samantha Bax

Intermittent Fasting For Women Over 50
Samantha Bax

Copyright 2023 © Prose Books LLC

All rights reserved.

No portion of this book may be reproduced without written permission from the publisher or author except as permitted by U.S. copyright law.

This publication is designed to provide accurate and authoritative information regarding the subject matter covered. It is sold with the understanding that neither the author nor the publisher is engaged in rendering legal, investment, accounting, or other professional services.

While the publisher and author have used their best efforts in preparing this book, they make no representations or warranties with respect to the accuracy or completeness of the contents of this book and specifically disclaim any implied warranties of merchantability or fitness for a particular purpose. Sales representatives or written sales materials may create or extend no warranty.

The advice and strategies contained herein may not be suitable for your situation. You should consult with a professional when appropriate. Neither the publisher nor the author shall be liable for any loss of profit or other commercial damages, including but not limited to special, incidental, consequential, personal, or other damages.

Prose Books
Prose Books LLC
Merrimack, NH 03054 USA
email: info@prosebooks.us

Table of Contents:

Table of Contents: iii
Foreward iv
Preface vi
Chapter 1: Understanding Intermittent Fasting 1
Chapter 2: Health Challenges for Women Over 50 4
Chapter 3: The Science Behind Intermittent Fasting 7
Chapter 4: Getting Started with Intermittent Fasting 10
Chapter 5: Health Benefits of Intermittent Fasting 13
Chapter 6: Different Intermittent Fasting Methods 16
Chapter 7: Integrating Lifestyle Changes 19
Chapter 8: Sustainable Weight Loss Strategies 23
Chapter 9: Harnessing Intermittent Fasting for Metabolic Reset 27
Chapter 10: A Blueprint for a Fulfilling Life Beyond 50 31
Chapter 11: Breaking the Fast - Breakfast Delights 37
Chapter 12: Midday Meals - Lunch Favorites 51
Chapter 13: The Heart of Dining - Main Course Creations 65
Chapter 14: Guilt-Free Pleasures - Snacks & Desserts 80
Chapter15: Complementary Flavors - Side Recipes 94
Bonus Recipes (with corresponding Chapter as reference) 108
Conclusion: Your Transformative Journey Begins Now 137
Appendix: Frequently Asked Questions about Intermittent Fasting 140
About The Author 143
Other Books by Samantha Bax 145
Thank You 148
BONUS: FREE Meal-Planner 149

Foreward

This book serves as a resource providing insights into how intermittent fasting can revitalize your metabolism, boost energy levels, and enhance memory while promoting a healthy lifestyle. Its purpose is to motivate you to take charge of your health and not allow age-related issues to dictate your life.

"Intermittent Fasting for Women Over 50" is a guide specifically tailored to women who are entering the stages of life. It addresses the health challenges and bodily changes that are often associated with this phase, including those related to menopause and aging.

What sets ***"Intermittent Fasting for Women Over 50"*** apart is its ability to demystify the world of weight loss advice. Drawing from experiences and overcoming marketing tactics, the author shares genuine and relatable perspectives.

Inside the book, you'll find:

- Stories and testimonials on the effectiveness of fasting.
- An introductory overview of fasting principles.
- Scientific explanations that support fasting.
- Guidance for successfully implementing intermittent fasting.
- A comprehensive list of health benefits associated with fasting.
- Methods of intermittent fasting are suitable for different lifestyles.
- Tips on incorporating lifestyle changes alongside fasting.

Discover strategies to overcome the challenges of dieting and achieve weight loss. Learn techniques to utilize fasting for resetting your metabolism.

This book goes beyond being a diet guide; it serves as a blueprint for embracing a fulfilling and healthier life after reaching the age of 50. It inspires readers to seize every moment, take control of their well-being, and embark on life's journey with renewed energy and enthusiasm.

"Intermittent Fasting for Women Over 50" extends an invitation to embark on a journey towards achieving health and happiness.

Preface

Embracing Your Golden Years

Introduction to the Book's Purpose and Message

Welcome to an adventure that extends far beyond simple recipes and ingredients. Within the pages of this book, we extend an invitation for you to embrace the years of your life and discover the transformative power that lies within food, flavors, and the art of cooking. Our intention is to inspire you with every turn of the page, encouraging you to create meals that nourish both your body and soul while cherishing each moment life has bestowed upon you.

This publication is more than a compilation of recipes; it stands as a testament to celebrating life, love, and the pure joy found in cooking. We firmly believe that the kitchen serves as a sanctuary where time seems to slow down, allowing for the enchanting alchemy of flavors to occur. It's a space where memories are formed, traditions are upheld, and new ones are born. As we embark on this chapter in our lives, we have been gifted with an opportunity to embrace our passions, fully explore territories, and create a legacy that future generations will hold dear.

A Personal Tale: Samantha Bax's Story Behind Writing this Book

As I take on the role of author for this piece of literature, I feel incredibly honored to share not only my personal journey but also the motivations that lie at its core. To me, the world of cuisine has always served as my refuge—a place where solace is found and my creativity flourishes.

It all started with a passion for the art of cooking, a love that has grown within me since I was young. However, unlike chefs and culinary experts who seek the spotlight, I've always preferred to stay behind the scenes, focusing on my words and the enchanting culinary experiences they portray.

My journey into the realm of cookbooks was an endeavor fueled by this profound love for food and culinary skills. It emerged from a desire to share my wisdom encounters and the flavors that have influenced my life. Through my writing, I aspire to transport you to a place where flavors gracefully dance on your taste buds and where cooking becomes an expression of oneself.

I embarked on this writing adventure, firmly believing that food can nourish not only our bodies but our souls. My hope is that as you embrace your years and immerse yourself in the culinary escapades found within these pages, you will discover the immense joy and fulfillment that cooking can provide.

Creating this book has been an act of devotion, serving as evidence of my dedication as a wordsmith in the world. I have poured every ounce of my passion into every word written, every recipe crafted, and every story shared. My writing style is characterized by its precision, clarity, and the touch of elegance it carries. Its purpose is to guide you through the world of the kitchen, igniting your imagination and inspiring your creativity.

Why have I chosen to remain anonymous? It's not because I lack pride in my work; rather, it's a decision to let the recipes and stories take the stage. In a world that constantly craves exposure and oversharing, I firmly believe in the power of words and recipes to speak for themselves. I want my creation's essence to shine without any distractions from a persona. By being an enigma, my intention is to emphasize the importance of the legacy we leave behind. The impact we can make without seeking personal recognition.

As you embark on this journey, I wholeheartedly encourage you to approach each recipe with a mind and a willingness to explore new flavors. Embrace the process of creation, experiment with ingredients, and infuse each dish with your touch.

Remember that cooking isn't about nourishing our bodies; it's about nourishing our souls well—connecting with loved ones and creating memories that will endure for a lifetime.

Within the following pages, you will discover a collection of recipes, each one showcasing my deep passion and expertise. From family favorites to exciting and innovative culinary trends, these dishes offer a wide variety of flavors to suit every palate. However, they hold more significance than that. They extend an invitation to celebrate life, relish the present moment, and warmly embrace the golden years.

As you immerse yourself in the chapters, always remember that the true joy of writing lies not in basking in the limelight but in knowing that our words have enriched the lives of home cooks. I sincerely hope that each recipe you try draws you closer to your legacy and infuses your own story with delightful flavors.

Together, let us embark on this journey while embracing our golden years with open hearts and an unwavering passion for the art of cooking. May these pages ignite inspiration within you, fuel your creativity endlessly, and fill your days with the pleasure of sharing a meal with your loved ones.

Welcome to a world brimming with flavors, unforgettable experiences, and the transformative power found in embracing the life phase.

Chapter 1: Understanding Intermittent Fasting

Overview of Intermittent Fasting Principles

In the years, intermittent fasting has gained a lot of attention as an effective way to improve health, facilitate weight loss, and enhance overall well-being. It's important to note that intermittent fasting is not another diet; it is actually a practice deeply rooted in our human evolutionary history. In this chapter, we will delve into the core principles of fasting, understand how it functions, and explore its advantages. Moreover, we will discuss approaches to fasting so that you can choose the one that aligns best with your lifestyle and goals.

Explanation of How It Works and Its Benefits

Intermittent fasting, at its core, involves alternating between periods of fasting and eating. Unlike diets that focus on what you eat, intermittent fasting focuses on when you eat. By extending the fasting period that occurs during sleep, intermittent fasting takes advantage of the body's metabolic and hormonal responses to optimize health.

When we consume food, our bodies break it down. Convert it into energy through digestion and metabolism. During this process, insulin is released to regulate blood sugar levels. Insulin also plays a role in storing energy as fat. However, during periods of fasting, insulin levels decrease, which prompts the body to utilize stored fat for energy needs. This physiological response is crucial for the benefits associated with fasting.

One of the advantages of fasting is its ability to support weight loss and improve body composition. By creating a calorie deficit during the fasting period, the body burns stored fat over time, leading to weight loss. Additionally, intermittent fasting has been demonstrated to preserve muscle mass while reducing body fat, improving the quality of weight loss.

In addition to weight loss benefits, intermittent fasting offers a range of health advantages. Studies have shown that this approach enhances insulin sensitivity and reduces the risk of developing type 2 diabetes.

Furthermore, intermittent fasting has been found to support autophagy, a process that aids in the elimination of cells and proteins. This, in turn, reduces the likelihood of developing ailments like cancer and Alzheimer's disease. Moreover, by mitigating inflammation and oxidative stress levels, intermittent fasting can enhance well-being while also benefiting function.

Different Types of Intermittent Fasting Methods

Intermittent fasting is not a one-size-fits-all-all strategy. There are methods to choose from, allowing individuals to find a fasting schedule that suits their lifestyle and preferences. Here are some of the types of intermittent fasting:

Time Restricted Feeding (TRF): With TRF, you limit the hours in which you consume food each day. The 16:8 method, where you fast for 16 hours and restrict your eating window to 8 hours, is quite popular. This can be achieved by skipping breakfast and having your meal at noon and then finishing it by 8 pm.

Alternate Day Fasting (ADF): ADF involves alternating between days of fasting and regular eating days. On some days, you consume a number of calories or fast completely, while on regular eating days, you eat as you normally would.

5:2 Diet: In this method, you follow your diet for five days a week. Restrict your calorie intake to approximately 500 to 600 calories on two non-consecutive days.

24-Hour Fasting: With this approach, you fast for 24 hours twice a week. For instance, a scenario could be that you finish your dinner at 7 pm and then don't eat again until 7 pm the following day.

Ultimately, the effective way of practicing fasting will vary based on your personal preferences, schedule, and desired outcomes.

As you embark on your journey with fasting, it's important to remember to listen to your body, stay properly hydrated, and prioritize eating dense foods during your designated eating periods. In the chapters, we will delve into each fasting method in detail, equipping you with the tools and knowledge to optimize the advantages of intermittent fasting.

Understanding the principles, mechanisms, and various approaches to fasting is the first step toward fully harnessing its potential. As you continue reading, you'll develop a deeper comprehension of how intermittent fasting can truly transform your health and overall well-being.

Chapter 2: Health Challenges for Women Over 50

When women reach their forties, they often come across a range of health issues that are specific to this stage of life. Menopause and the aging process bring about changes in a woman's body, which can affect her overall well-being. In this chapter, we'll explore the topic of the health challenges encountered during menopause and aging, focusing on how hormonal changes, physical transformations, and a decrease in metabolism can have an impact. By gaining an understanding of these challenges, women can proactively take measures to maintain their health and enhance their quality of life.

Discussion on the Unique Health Challenges Faced during Menopause and Aging

Menopause, which typically happens between the ages of 45 and 55, signifies the conclusion of a woman's ability to have children. It is an event that involves a notable decline in hormone production, especially estrogen and progesterone. These changes in hormones can result in emotional symptoms, such as sudden bursts of heat, excessive sweating at night, fluctuating moods, dryness in the vaginal area, and disruptions in sleep patterns.

The effects of changes during menopause go beyond these symptoms. For instance, estrogen plays a role in maintaining bone density. As its levels decline, women face an increased risk of developing osteoporosis—a condition characterized by brittle bones. Additionally, the aging process contributes to a decrease in muscle mass, which further raises the chance of falls and fractures.

Apart from bone health concerns, hormonal changes also impact well-being. Estrogen offers protection to the heart by maintaining blood vessels and regulating cholesterol levels. However, with its decline during menopause, women become more susceptible to diseases like heart attacks and strokes. Therefore, it becomes essential for women over 50 to prioritize a healthy lifestyle by engaging in exercise routines, adopting a balanced diet, and scheduling routine health checkups.

As women age further into menopause, they face challenges related to body changes and metabolism slowdown. Many women experience weight gain during this phase, predominantly around the abdomen area.

The changes in body composition that occur with age are influenced by shifts and the decrease in muscle mass and metabolic rate. This can make it more difficult for women to lose weight and maintain a body weight.

Additionally, as metabolism slows down, the body's response to food and nutrient absorption may be affected. Women over 50 need to pay attention to their diet as their nutrient requirements may change. Nutrients like calcium and vitamin D become more crucial for maintaining bone health. Therefore, they need to include a variety of foods in their diet to meet their evolving needs.

Addressing the Health Challenges

Despite the challenges that come with menopause and aging, there are strategies that women can adopt to minimize their impact and maintain health. First and foremost, seeking guidance is crucial. Consulting with a healthcare provider can help identify risks. Develop personalized strategies to address specific health concerns.

One common approach to managing symptoms is hormone replacement therapy (HRT). By supplementing declining hormone levels, HRT can alleviate flashes, improve sleep quality, and protect bone health. However, the decision to pursue HRT should be made in consultation with a healthcare professional, taking into account an individual's history and potential risks.

Adopting a lifestyle plays a role in managing the health challenges associated with menopause and aging. Regular exercise, including weight-bearing activities, helps maintain bone density, manage weight, and improve health. Engaging in strength training exercises also combats muscle loss while promoting strength and balance.

A nutritious diet is equally important. A balanced approach that includes grains, lean proteins, fruits, vegetables, and healthy fats provides the necessary nutrients for overall health support. Paying attention to calcium and vitamin D intake is particularly crucial for maintaining bones. Additionally, reducing the consumption of processed foods along with alcohol and caffeine intake can help alleviate symptoms.

In Chapter 2, we've explored the health issues that women over 50 encounter as they go through menopause and aging. The changes in hormones, body, and metabolism during this phase can have an impact on a woman's well-being. However, with the knowledge and support, women can successfully navigate these challenges. By seeking advice, adopting a lifestyle, and making appropriate adjustments to their diet and exercise routines, women can maintain good health, energy levels, and quality of life well into their 50s and beyond.

Chapter 3: The Science Behind Intermittent Fasting

In the years, intermittent fasting (IF) has become widely recognized as a trendy eating habit. Apart from its connection to weight loss, IF is believed to offer health advantages on both metabolic and cellular levels. This section investigates the reasoning behind fasting by examining research results and studies that validate its efficacy. By exploring the benefits it provides to our metabolism and cells, we can better comprehend why intermittent fasting has captivated the interest of scientists and health enthusiasts alike.

Effects of Intermittent Fasting on the Body

Intermittent fasting brings about a series of changes in our bodies that have an impact on our well-being. One notable effect is the decrease in insulin levels during the fasting period, which in turn promotes the burning and utilization of stored energy. Consequently, intermittent fasting has been linked to weight loss and improved body composition.

Moreover, intermittent fasting encourages a process called autophagy, where damaged or dysfunctional components are recycled and eliminated. This cleansing mechanism is upregulated during the fasting state, effectively removing proteins and damaged organelles. Research suggests that this cellular rejuvenation process may reduce the risk of diseases such as Alzheimer's and Parkinson's.

Research Findings and Studies Supporting Effectiveness

Numerous studies have delved into the impacts of fasting on health and well-being, presenting strong evidence to support its effectiveness. For instance, Varady et al. conducted a study that showed how alternate-day fasting resulted in reductions in body weight, body fat, and insulin levels among adults. Similarly, Harvie et al. discovered that intermittent energy restriction led to weight loss and improved insulin sensitivity in women with a risk of breast cancer. These findings underscore the benefits of fasting for weight management and metabolic health.

Moreover, intermittent fasting holds promise for extending lifespan and promoting longevity. A study conducted on mice by Mattson et al. It was discovered that intermittent fasting contributed to increased lifespan and a lower incidence of age-related diseases like cancer and diabetes. While further research is necessary to determine if similar effects manifest in humans, these findings suggest that intermittent fasting may offer the potential for promoting aging.

Understanding the Metabolic and Cellular Benefits

Intermittent fasting offers benefits to our metabolism and cellular health, going beyond weight loss and disease prevention. One key factor behind these benefits is hormesis, where mild stressors prompt our cells to adapt and function better. During fasting periods, the body experiences a stress response that triggers cellular pathways, including the activation of sirtuins and AMP-activated protein kinase (AMPK). These pathways enhance our cells' resilience, improve energy metabolism, and provide protection against age-related diseases.

Moreover, intermittent fasting stimulates the formation of mitochondria within our cells through a process called biogenesis. Mitochondria are like powerhouses for our cells; they produce energy. By increasing the number and efficiency of mitochondria, intermittent fasting boosts energy production. Supports optimal cellular function.

In Chapter 3, we've delved into the explanations for how intermittent fasting affects our bodies. By reducing insulin levels, promoting autophagy (cleaning), and triggering hormesis (the body's response), intermittent fasting activates various metabolic and cellular pathways that contribute to its numerous health benefits. Research findings and studies have provided evidence in support of its effectiveness in weight loss disease prevention. Even potentially extending lifespan. Understanding these mechanisms lays the groundwork for recognizing the potential of fasting as an approach to enhance overall health and well-being.

Chapter 4: Getting Started with Intermittent Fasting

Intermittent fasting has become quite popular in recent years because of its many health advantages and effectiveness in managing weight. Suppose you are thinking about embracing fasting as a way of life. In that case, this chapter will provide you with guidance on how to begin and successfully incorporate it. By following the step-by-step instructions, discovering the fasting schedule that suits your lifestyle, and making use of tips, you will be able to gradually adapt to the fasting routine and enjoy the benefits that intermittent fasting offers.

Step-by-Step Guide on Implementing Intermittent Fasting Successfully

Get Informed: Before you start your fasting journey, it's essential to educate yourself about the fasting methods available and how they can fit into your lifestyle. Take some time to research fasting protocols, like the 16/8 method, the 5:2 diet, or alternate-day fasting. Consider which one aligns best with your goals and preferences.

Take It Slow: Intermittent fasting requires a period of adjustment for your body to adapt. It's recommended that you begin fasting periods, such as 12 to 14 hours, and gradually increase the duration over time. This gradual approach will allow your body to get used to fasting and minimize any discomfort.

Choose Your Fasting Window: Decide on the times for your fasting and eating windows that suit both your routine and personal preferences. The popular approach is a 16-hour fasting window followed by an 8-hour eating window. Feel free to adjust these times based on what works best for you. Experiment with schedules until you find the one that fits seamlessly into your life.

Stay Hydrated: It's crucial to keep yourself hydrated during your fasting period. Make sure to drink water, herbal tea, or other non-caloric beverages in order to maintain hydration levels and help curb any hunger pangs you may experience.

Finding the Right Fasting Schedule for Your Lifestyle

Think about your routine: Take into consideration your work schedule, social commitments, and personal preferences when deciding on your fasting schedule. If you enjoy having breakfast with your family or dinner with friends, adjust your fasting and eating windows accordingly.

Pay attention to what your body tells you: Observe how your body reacts to fasting schedules. Some people may find it easier to fast in the morning, while others may prefer skipping dinner. Experiment with fasting and eating windows until you discover the schedule that suits the needs of your body and allows you to maintain consistency.

Tips and Tricks to Ease into the Fasting Routine

Gradually Decrease Meal Frequency: If you currently have three meals a day, consider reducing it to two meals before starting to fast. This will help your body adapt to periods without eating.

Prioritize Nutrient-Rich Foods: When you break your fast, focus on consuming foods that are packed with vitamins, minerals, and macronutrients. Choose grains, lean proteins, fruits, vegetables, and healthy fats to effectively nourish your body.

Managing Hunger and Cravings: Keeping yourself busy with activities can be useful in managing hunger and cravings during the fasting period. Engage in activities like reading, exercising, or spending quality time with loved ones. Additionally, sipping on calorie beverages such as coffee or herbal tea in small amounts can help control your appetite.

Find Support: Starting fasting might be challenging at first, especially if you're accustomed to eating. Look for a support system such as a friend, family member, or online community where you can share experiences, seek advice, and stay motivated throughout your fasting journey.

Remember that intermittent fasting is a lifestyle change that requires some adjustment time. Be patient with yourself. Don't let occasional setbacks discourage you.

Achieving success in experiencing the benefits of fasting requires consistency and perseverance. By following this guide, you can find the fasting schedule that suits your lifestyle and gradually incorporate strategies to adopt the fasting routine. This will lead you towards embracing fasting as a rewarding lifestyle choice.

Chapter 5: Health Benefits of Intermittent Fasting

Intermittent fasting has become increasingly popular in recent years due to its health benefits. In this chapter, we will explore the range of advantages that intermittent fasting offers, such as increased metabolism, enhanced energy levels, enhanced cognitive function, and positive effects on concerns related to aging.

Enhanced Metabolism: One of the perks of fasting is its ability to boost metabolism. By limiting the hours in which we consume calories, our bodies are encouraged to utilize energy reserves. This process, known as autophagy, promotes rejuvenation. Supports overall metabolic health and weight management.

Heightened Energy Levels: Research indicates that intermittent fasting can enhance energy levels by improving function. During periods of fasting, our bodies adapt to using stored fat as a source of fuel. This leads to increased energy levels and better physical performance throughout the day, ultimately aiding productivity and overall well-being.

Improved Cognitive Function: Emerging evidence suggests that intermittent fasting can have effects on brain health and cognitive function. Fasting triggers the release of brain-derived factor (BDNF), a protein that facilitates growth and connectivity among nerve cells. As a result, overall brain function is enhanced.

Moreover, intermittent fasting has been linked to memory, concentration, and mental sharpness, making it a promising approach for maintaining well-being.

Exploring the Positive Effects on Aging-related Concerns: Aging is a process influenced by factors, including oxidative stress and inflammation. Intermittent fasting shows promise in mitigating these age-related concerns, potentially promoting a healthier life. By reducing stress, fasting shields cells from damage caused by radicals, thus lowering the risk of chronic diseases like cardiovascular disease, diabetes, and certain cancers.

Furthermore, intermittent fasting triggers cellular repair mechanisms such as autophagy and DNA repair that help counteract the effects of aging. These processes eliminate malfunctioning proteins and cellular waste material while promoting regeneration and overall rejuvenation. Intermittent fasting has also demonstrated its ability to decrease inflammation markers like C reactive protein (CRP) and interleukin 6 (IL 6), which are commonly associated with age-related diseases.

Apart from its impact on aging itself, intermittent fasting may provide benefits for age-related decline and neurodegenerative diseases. Studies involving animals have shown that intermittent fasting can safeguard against conditions such as Alzheimer's and Parkinson's disease by reducing the accumulation of proteins while enhancing function.

While more research is still needed, these findings present promising insights into how intermittent fasting may contribute to promoting aging.

In conclusion, this chapter has explored a list of health benefits that come with fasting. These include improved metabolism, increased energy levels, enhanced cognitive function, and positive effects on age-related concerns. Intermittent fasting has proven itself to be a tool for well-being. By incorporating fasting into a lifestyle, individuals can take advantage of its numerous benefits and optimize their physical and mental health. In the chapter, we will delve deeper into methods of intermittent fasting and provide practical tips for successful implementation.

Chapter 6: Different Intermittent Fasting Methods

In-depth Explanation of Various Intermittent Fasting Protocols

Intermittent fasting has become extremely popular in recent years due to its many health benefits and effectiveness in managing weight. In this chapter, we will explore methods of fasting, aiming to provide a thorough understanding of each approach. Furthermore, we will evaluate how suitable these methods are for women over the age of 50, taking into consideration the factors that may impact their fasting experience.

16/8 Method:

The 16/8 method is a commonly used fasting approach. It involves fasting for 16 hours and limiting eating to an 8-hour window each day. This method usually allows for two to three meals during the eating period. The 16/8 method is relatively easy to follow as it aligns with the fasting time and allows individuals to skip breakfast if desired.

This approach is particularly suitable for women who are over 50 years old as it offers flexibility and supports a transition into fasting. However, it's important to note that women in this age group may experience changes that can affect their response to fasting. Therefore, it is recommended to monitor any changes in mood, energy levels, or overall well-being while practicing the 16/8 method.

Alternate-Day Fasting:

Alternate-day fasting is a method where you alternate between days of fasting and days of eating. During the fasting days, people usually consume fewer calories than 500. On the eating days, they can stick to their eating habits. This approach might be a bit challenging for beginners because of the periods of fasting. It has shown promising results in terms of weight loss and overall health improvement.

For women who are over 50 years alternate-day fasting might not be a suitable choice, especially if they are dealing with hormonal imbalances or other health issues. The nature of this method can lead to increased stress levels and potential disruptions in hormone regulation. It recommended that women in this age group consult with healthcare before considering alternate-day fasting.

5:2 Method:

The 5:2 approach involves following an eating pattern for five days each week. Then, restricting calorie intake to around 500 to 600 calories on the remaining two days. This method combines the benefits of fasting with a bit of flexibility throughout the week. It's important to spread out the fasting days across the week to avoid fasting days.

For women over 50, the 5:2 method can be an option as it provides a strict fasting routine. It allows for balancing calorie intake and meeting nutrient requirements, which is particularly important for women in this age group who may have specific dietary needs. However, it's crucial to prioritize well-being and make adjustments to the fasting protocol if needed.

Other Intermittent Fasting Protocols:

In addition to the methods mentioned earlier, there are intermittent fasting approaches that have their own unique variations. For example, there is the Eat Stop Eat method, where you fast for 24 hours twice a week, and the Warrior Diet, which allows calorie intake during the day and unrestricted eating at night.

When considering these protocols for women over 50, it's important to approach them with caution. The hormonal changes that occur during menopause can affect metabolism, energy levels, and overall health. Therefore, personalized adjustments may be needed to ensure results and address any concerns.

Intermittent fasting offers a variety of protocols that can be customized based on needs and preferences. While the 16/8 method and the 5:2 method are generally suitable for women over 50, it's crucial to consider health conditions and consult healthcare professionals before starting any fasting regimen. By understanding the fasting methods and their potential effects on women, over 50 individuals can make informed decisions that align with their specific needs and goals.

Chapter 7: Integrating Lifestyle Changes

O In our path to achieving a more satisfying life, we've delved into the advantages and complexities of fasting. Now, let us explore the world of lifestyle adjustments and learn how we can effortlessly blend them into our fasting routine. In this section, we'll discuss advice for integrating lifestyle changes while practicing intermittent fasting. Additionally, we'll cover exercise recommendations specifically tailored for women over 50 as the crucial significance of self-care and stress management. By embracing these changes, we can improve our well-being. Please make the most out of our fasting journey.

Section 1: Tips for Incorporating Healthy Lifestyle Changes Alongside Intermittent Fasting

Taking an approach is crucial when it comes to incorporating lifestyle changes. Instead of overwhelming ourselves with changes all at once, it's better to focus on making one change at a time. This allows for adaptation. Increases the chances of successfully integrating it into your fasting routine.

One unique aspect of fasting is that it provides an opportunity to develop a relationship with food. Embrace mindful eating by savoring each bite, choosing foods that are packed with nutrients, and paying attention to your hunger and fullness cues. Practicing mindfulness in this way enhances the effectiveness of fasting and promotes long-term healthy habits.

Hydration plays a role in maintaining health, especially during fasting periods. Make sure to drink plenty of water throughout the day, even while you're fasting. You can make your hydration more enjoyable by infusing water with flavors like lemon or cucumber.

To meet your body's needs, prioritize consuming a balanced diet that includes plenty of fruits, vegetables, lean proteins, whole grains, and healthy fats. By providing your body with nutrients through this nourishing diet, you'll optimize your fasting experience. Improve your overall well-being.

Section 2: Exercise Recommendations for Women over 50

Exercise plays a role in maintaining a healthy lifestyle, regardless of age or gender. Women aged 50 and above particularly benefit from the activity, offering advantages such as enhanced bone density, cardiovascular health, and mental well-being. Here are some exercise recommendations tailored specifically for women in this age group;

1. Cardiovascular Exercises: Engaging in activities like walking, swimming, cycling, or dancing can greatly improve heart health and endurance. It is recommended to aim for 150 minutes of moderate-intensity aerobic activity per week or 75 minutes of vigorous-intensity activity.

2. Strength Training: Including strength training exercises that involve weights or resistance bands is essential for preserving muscle mass and bone density. Focus on all muscle groups, including the legs, arms, back, chest, and core. Aim for two or more sessions per week while allowing rest and recovery time between sessions.

3. Flexibility and Balance: As we grow older, flexibility and balance become increasingly important. Exercises such as yoga, tai chi, or Pilates are incorporated into your routine to enhance flexibility, balance, and posture, as well as promote relaxation and mental well-being.

4. Listen to Your Body: Always pay close attention to your body's signals during exercise to avoid overexertion or injury.

Remember that these recommendations are specifically designed for women over 50. It's always advisable to consult with a healthcare before starting any new exercise regimen.

If you feel any discomfort or pain, it's important to adjust or select more suitable exercises for your abilities and specific needs. Before beginning any exercise routine, it is always advisable to consult with a healthcare professional.

Section 3: Emphasizing the Importance of Self-Care and Stress Management

Incorporating lifestyle adjustments and intermittent fasting can have an impact. It is equally important to prioritize taking care of yourself and managing stress. Here are some strategies to help you navigate through the challenges.

Quality Sleep: Make sure you're getting sleep each night to support your body's natural healing processes. Establish a soothing bedtime routine. Stick to a sleep schedule. Avoid using devices before bed and create a peaceful and comfortable sleeping environment.

Mindfulness and Stress Relief: Integrate stress reduction techniques into your routine, such as meditation, deep breathing exercises, or engaging in activities that bring you joy. Practicing mindfulness can help reduce stress levels, enhance focus, and contribute to well-being.

Social Connections: Foster meaningful. Maintain a support system. Participate in activities that encourage connections, whether it's spending time with loved ones or joining community groups aligned with your interests.

Time for Yourself: Set aside time for self-care activities that recharge your mind, body, and soul. This could involve pursuing hobbies, enjoying relaxing baths, reading books, or indulging in activities that bring you joy.

By incorporating these self-care practices and stress management techniques alongside fasting and lifestyle changes, you'll create an approach to well-being that maximizes your overall potential.

Incorporating habits into your lifestyle while practicing fasting can create a powerful synergy that can bring about significant positive changes in your overall well-being, encompassing physical, mental, and emotional aspects. By adopting these changes, including exercise routines designed specifically for women over 50 and prioritizing self-care and stress management, you will unleash the potential of your fasting journey. Embrace this combination. Explore the incredible rewards that await you on the path toward a healthier and more satisfying life.

Chapter 8: Sustainable Weight Loss Strategies

When it comes to achieving lasting weight loss, it's important to have the mindset and use strategies that go beyond quick fixes. This chapter is designed to help you navigate the challenges of yo-yo dieting, offer tips for weight loss through fasting, and assist you in developing positive habits and a mindset that will lead to long-term success.

Guidance on Avoiding the Pitfalls of Yo-Yo Dieting

Yo-yo dieting, also known as weight cycling, is when you repeatedly lose weight, gain it back, and then start the cycle again. This type of approach can be harmful to your mental health, making it difficult to achieve long-term weight loss. To avoid falling into this pattern, here are some important guidelines to keep in mind;

1. Say no to quick fixes; Sustainable weight loss is a journey rather than a sprint. Avoid crash diets or extreme measures that promise results. Instead, focus on making sustainable changes to your eating habits and lifestyle.

2. **Embrace balance:** Opt for a rounded diet that includes a variety of foods with nutrients. Avoid diets that eliminate entire food groups, as they may lead to nutritional deficiencies and cravings.

3. **Portion control matters:** Be mindful of portion sizes and practice eating. Engage all your senses while enjoying your meals, savor each bite, and stop eating when you feel comfortably satisfied. This mindful approach will help you develop a relationship with food.

4. Seek advice: Consider consulting with a registered dietitian or nutritionist who can provide guidance tailored to your specific needs and goals. They can assist you in creating a sustainable plan that fits well with your lifestyle.

Tips for Achieving Sustainable Weight Loss with Intermittent Fasting

Intermittent fasting has become increasingly popular as a method for achieving weight loss results. By incorporating periods of fasting into your routine, you can experience its benefits while maintaining a healthy lifestyle. Here are some tips to help you make fasting work effectively.

1. Choose the fasting method that suits you: There are fasting methods available, such as the 16/8 method or alternate-day fasting. Experiment with approaches to find the one that best fits your schedule and preferences.

2. Start gradually: If you're new to fasting, it's recommended to begin with periods of fasting and gradually increase the duration as your body adapts. This approach helps minimize side effects and allows for a transition.

3. Stay well hydrated: It's crucial to keep yourself hydrated during the fasting periods by drinking water, herbal teas, or other non-caloric beverages. Maintaining hydration helps control hunger and supports well-being.

4. Prioritize meals: When breaking your fast, focus on consuming whole foods that are rich in nutrients to ensure you meet your nutritional requirements. Include proteins, healthy fats, fiber-rich carbohydrates, and ample amounts of fruits and vegetables in your meals.

Mindset Shifts and Positive Habits to Support Long-term Success

Achieving lasting and healthy weight loss goes beyond focusing on diet and exercise. It involves developing a mindset and adopting habits. Here are some mindset shifts and habits that can help support your long-term success.

1. Set goals: Fixating solely on the number, on the scale, aim for achievable goals like improving your fitness level, increasing your energy, or reducing waist circumference. Celebrate victories along the way, not those related to weight.

2. Practice self-compassion: Be kind to yourself throughout your weight loss journey. Avoid criticizing yourself when setbacks occur; instead, learn from them. Use them as motivation to keep going. Patience is key, and every bit of progress is worth acknowledging.

3. Build a support system: Surround yourself with individuals who share goals or have successfully achieved sustainable weight loss themselves. You can join communities, find accountability partners, or consider joining fitness or weight loss groups.

4. Prioritize self-care: Make self-care a part of your routine that you don't compromise on. Ensure you get to sleep effectively, manage stress levels, and incorporate activities you enjoy into your daily life. Taking care of your emotional well-being is crucial for long-term success.

By implementing these mindset shifts and habits into your journey towards weight loss, you'll be setting yourself up for lasting success in a holistic way.

Conclusion

To achieve long-term weight loss, it is important to adopt a holistic approach that includes well-informed strategies, a positive mindset, and healthy habits. Instead of falling into the trap of yo-yo dieting, you should focus on effectively incorporating fasting and cultivating the right mindset. By doing you will be able to not lose weight but also make a lasting transformation in your life. Keep in mind that this journey is not about rushing through it; rather, it requires a commitment to your well-being.

Chapter 9: Harnessing Intermittent Fasting for Metabolic Reset

Techniques to Reset Your Metabolism and Improve Overall Health

Intermittent fasting has become increasingly popular because of its advantages in terms of metabolic health and weight control. By timing periods of fasting and eating, people can harness their body's ability to burn fat, increase energy levels, and enhance overall well-being. In this chapter, we will delve into methods to reset your metabolism successfully and improve your health through intermittent fasting.

Start with the Basics: Time-Restricted Eating

A straightforward and easily achievable way to practice fasting is through time-restricted eating (TRE). This method entails restricting your eating period to a number of hours each day, typically ranging from 8 to 10 hours. By condensing your meals into a timeframe, you give your body the opportunity to enter a fasting state for the rest of the day. This promotes burning. Enhances metabolic efficiency. To optimize the advantages, it's important to align your eating window with your body's rhythm.

Alternate-Day Fasting: A Powerful Tool

If you're looking for a method, you might consider alternate-day fasting (ADF) as a viable approach to reset your metabolism. ADF involves alternating between fasting days and days when you can eat normally. During the fasting days, you significantly reduce your caloric intake to around 500 to 600 calories. On the other hand, feasting days allow you to consume food without any restrictions. ADF has been found to have effects on insulin sensitivity, cellular repair processes, and fat oxidation, making it an effective tool for resetting your metabolism.

Extended Fasting: Unlocking the Power of Autophagy

Although it can be more challenging, practicing fasting has the potential to bring about improvements in metabolic function and overall health. Extended fasting involves abstaining from food for periods exceeding 24 hours, ranging from 36 to 72 hours or longer. During this time, your body depletes its glycogen stores. Starts relying on stored fat for energy. Additionally, extended fasting triggers a process called autophagy, which is a self-cleansing mechanism that eliminates damaged molecules and rejuvenates cells. This does not help with metabolic reset. Also supports cellular health and longevity.

Maximizing the Benefits of Intermittent Fasting for Optimal Results

To maximize the advantages of fasting, it's important to focus on key factors:

1. Balanced Nutrition: While intermittent fasting doesn't restrict any food groups, maintaining a balanced diet is crucial for overall health. Prioritize nutrient foods such as fruits, vegetables, lean proteins, and healthy fats during your eating windows. These choices will provide your body with fuel. Support optimal metabolic function.

2. Hydration: It's essential to stay properly hydrated both during fasting and eating periods. Drinking water helps support the body's natural detoxification processes, aids digestion, and maintains metabolism. Aim for 8 cups of water per day, and consider adding herbal teas or infused water for variety and additional health benefits.

3. Regular Exercise: Combining fasting with exercise can enhance the metabolic benefits even more. Engaging in a mix of exercises, strength training, and flexibility exercises during your eating periods contributes to building muscle mass while improving insulin sensitivity and overall metabolic rate. However, it's advisable to avoid workouts during fasting periods as your body may require more rest and recovery time.

Strategies for Breaking Through Weight Loss Plateaus

Although intermittent fasting is a method for losing weight, it's not uncommon to hit plateaus along the way. To overcome these plateaus and maximize weight loss, here are some strategies you can try.

1. Adjust Your Eating Window: If you've been sticking to an eating schedule, consider changing the duration or timing of your eating window. Sometimes, our bodies get used to a routine, so shaking things up can help jumpstart your metabolism.

2. Incorporate High-Intensity Interval Training (HIIT): HIIT workouts involve bursts of exercise followed by rest periods. Studies have shown that this type of workout boosts calorie burn and fat oxidation, making it an excellent addition to fasting.

3. Assess Your Caloric Intake: While counting calories isn't necessary with fasting, it can be beneficial to evaluate how many calories you're consuming overall. Make sure you're not overeating during your eating window, as this could hinder your weight loss progress.

In summary, intermittent fasting is a tool for resetting your metabolism and enhancing health. By incorporating techniques like time-restricted eating, alternate-day fasting, and extended fasting, you can tap into your body's ability to burn fat and optimize metabolic function.

Furthermore, to optimize the advantages of fasting, it is crucial to maintain a rounded diet, stay hydrated, and engage in regular physical activity. Come across any hurdles in your weight loss journey. You can try modifying your eating schedule by incorporating high-intensity interval training (HIIT) and assessing your calorie consumption. Intermittent fasting offers a customizable method that can be tailored to meet your requirements and aspirations, ultimately resulting in enhanced overall health and wellness.

Chapter 10: A Blueprint for a Fulfilling Life Beyond 50

Longevity, vitality, and happiness are not just aspirations limited to the young. They are timeless dreams that can be realized at any point in life beyond the age of 50. In this section, we will delve into the elements of embracing a healthier life in the latter half of your journey. By sharing motivational quotes, anecdotes, and actionable advice, we aim to provide you with a roadmap for living your life—a life filled with meaning, happiness, and overall wellness.

Focusing on Longevity, Vitality, and Happiness

Over time, our outlook on life can go through transformations. Our priorities. We discover a renewed sense of purpose. In this chapter, we encourage you to embrace this phase with the intention of concentrating on three fundamental aspects: long-lasting well-being, vibrancy, and genuine happiness.

Longevity

"Life is not merely living, but living in health." - Marcus Valerius Martialis

To ensure a healthy life, it is important to prioritize our mental well-being. This can be achieved through exercise, maintaining a diet, and getting enough sleep. Engaging in activities that promote strength, flexibility, and cardiovascular health is key. Consider practicing yoga, swimming, or even going for walks to keep your body energized and fit. Remember, it's never too late to start taking care of yourself.

In addition to taking care of our bodies, we should also focus on nurturing our minds through learning. Exploring interests, acquiring skills, and engaging in creative pursuits can greatly enhance cognitive function, memory retention, and overall mental well-being.

Vitality

"Life is not measured by the number of breaths we take, but by the moments that take our breath away." - Maya Angelou

Living a fulfilling life involves approaching each day with enthusiasm, passion, and a clear sense of purpose. It's important to maintain a mindset as it holds the key to unlocking our vitality. Surround yourself with uplifting individuals who inspire and motivate you, as their influence can greatly impact your well-being. Engage in activities that bring you joy and fulfillment, whether by rediscovering forgotten passions or exploring hobbies that ignite your spirit.

Another crucial aspect is cultivating gratitude for the abundance in your life. Take time to reflect on the experiences that have shaped you, the relationships that have enriched you, and the achievements that have brought you a sense of pride. By appreciating the moment and nurturing your relationships, you will infuse each day with a renewed sense of vitality.

Happiness

"The purpose of our lives is to be happy." - Dalai Lama

Finding happiness is not a state; rather, it is a decision. It comes from leading a fulfilling life, one that is enriched with relationships, personal development, and contentment. Embrace the strength of connections by nurturing bonds with loved ones, friends, and your community. Practice acts of kindness and selflessness because when we uplift others, we uplift ourselves.

As you journey through life after reaching the age of 50, prioritize your well-being. Take care of yourself by engaging in activities that promote relaxation and reduce stress. Cultivate mindfulness. Embrace a mindset of acceptance. Let go of regrets and appreciate the beauty found in each present moment.

Inspiring Quotes, Stories, and Tips for Living Your Best Life

Throughout history, there have been individuals who defied expectations and paved their own paths to fulfillment even after reaching the age of 50. The stories of these individuals serve as a source of inspiration, guiding us on our personal journeys. Let their wisdom shed light on your path.

One shining example is Grandma Moses, an artist who embarked on her painting career at the age of 70. Through her captivating masterpieces, she showed the world that it's never too late to pursue our passions.

Another inspiring story is that of Colonel Harland Sanders, who founded Kentucky Fried Chicken when he was 62 years old. His tale serves as a reminder that age should never hinder our spirit.

Then there's Fauja Singh, a centenarian who completed a marathon at the age of 101. His achievement shattered stereotypes and proved that age should never be seen as a barrier to pursuing challenges or accomplishing feats.

In addition to these stories, we also offer advice for living your best life beyond 50.

1. Prioritize self-care. Make time for activities that replenish your energy.

2. Surround yourself with supportive individuals who believe in your potential.

3. Embrace the power of gratitude by practicing it

4. Continuously seek opportunities for growth and lifelong learning.

5. Engage in exercise. Maintain a well-balanced diet.

Let these valuable insights serve as your compass as you embark on this chapter brimming with opportunities and personal fulfillment!

Within the confines of this chapter, we have delved into the principles behind embracing a life of satisfaction and well-being after reaching the age of 50. By prioritizing longevity, vitality, and happiness, we establish a groundwork for an existence filled with joy.

Through thought-provoking quotes, captivating stories, and practical advice, we equip you with a roadmap to lead your life during the latter half of your journey. As you progress forward, always remember that age holds no limitations. Embrace the potentials that lie ahead and craft a life that exceeds your wildest aspirations.

RECIPES

Chapter 11: Breaking the Fast - Breakfast Delights

This chapter introduces a variety of nutritious and fulfilling breakfast recipes that perfectly align with the intermittent fasting schedule. It includes dishes that are both energizing and satisfying, ensuring a strong start to the day. From protein-packed smoothies to hearty omelets, these recipes are designed to provide sustained energy without feeling too heavy.

Here are some delicious breakfast recipes for you to try.

Recipe 1: Almond Butter and Banana Smoothie. Start your day with a nutritious smoothie made with almond butter, ripe bananas, and a hint of cinnamon. It's quick, energizing and satisfying.

Recipe 2: Spinach and Feta Omelet. Enjoy a fluffy omelet filled with spinach, crumbled feta cheese, and a touch of garlic. This protein-rich dish also provides a dose of greens.

Recipe 3: Avocado Toast with Poached Eggs. Treat yourself to whole-grain toast topped with creamy avocado. Poached eggs. Sprinkle some flakes. Squeeze fresh lemon for an extra kick.

Recipe 4: Greek Yogurt Parfait with Mixed Berries. Indulge in layers of Greek yogurt, fresh mixed berries, and granola, all drizzled with honey. It's a satisfying breakfast option.

Recipe 5: Chia Seed Pudding with Mango. Enjoy a pudding made by soaking chia seeds in milk. Top it off with mango chunks. Sprinkle some coconut flakes for added flavor.

Recipe 6: Quinoa Breakfast Bowl. Warm up your morning with a bowl of quinoa mixed with sliced almonds, dried cranberries, and a touch of cinnamon. Serve it alongside a dollop of Greek yogurt for creaminess.

Recipe 7: Veggie Breakfast Burrito. Savor the goodness of this burrito filled with scrambled eggs, bell peppers, onions, and black beans wrapped in a wheat tortilla. It is packed full of flavor!

These recipes offer variety while providing options to start your day on the note. Here are a few delicious recipes you can try:

Recipe 8: Peanut Butter and Banana Overnight Oats: Start your day with an easy breakfast option. Mix creamy peanut butter sliced. Overnight oats for a grab-and-go meal.

Recipe 9: Smoked Salmon Bagel with Cream Cheese: Enjoy the timeless combination of smoked salmon and cream cheese on a whole-grain bagel. Add some capers and red onion for a touch of flavor.

Recipe 10: Baked Sweet Potato and Kale Hash: Create a hash by roasting potatoes, sautéing kale, and sprinkling it all with paprika. Top it off with a fried egg for added deliciousness.

Recipe 11: Blueberry Walnut Pancakes: Treat yourself to pancakes packed with blueberries and crunchy chopped walnuts. Serve them warm with maple syrup on the side.

Recipe 12: Cottage Cheese Pineapple Bowl: Kickstart your day with this light yet satisfying dish. Combine cottage cheese chunks of pineapple and a sprinkle of chia seeds for a protein breakfast option.

Recipe 1: Almond Butter and Banana Smoothie

Prep Time: 5 mins - No Cooking - Serves: 2

Ingredients:
2 ripe bananas
2 tablespoons almond butter
1 cup almond milk or milk of choice
1/2 teaspoon cinnamon
1 tablespoon honey or maple syrup (optional)
Ice cubes (optional)

Instructions:
1. In a blender, combine the bananas, almond butter, almond milk, cinnamon, and honey or maple syrup if using.
2. Add a few ice cubes if you prefer a colder smoothie.
3. Blend on high speed until the mixture is smooth and creamy.
4. Taste and adjust the sweetness or cinnamon to your liking.
5. Pour the smoothie into glasses and serve immediately for a refreshing and energizing drink.

Nutritional Facts:
- Calories: 250
- Total Fat: 11g
- Total Carbs: 36g
- Fiber: 5g
- Net Carbs: 31g
- Protein: 6g

__Cooking Tip:__ For a thicker smoothie, you can add a scoop of Greek yogurt or use frozen bananas. To boost the nutritional content, consider adding a tablespoon of chia seeds or a scoop of your favorite protein powder.

Recipe 2: Spinach and Feta Omelet

Prep Time: 5 mins - Cooking Time: 10 mins - Serves: 1

Ingredients:
2 large eggs
1 tablespoon milk or water
Salt and pepper to taste
1 tablespoon olive oil
1 clove garlic, minced
1 cup fresh spinach leaves
1/4 cup feta cheese, crumbled
Optional: Fresh herbs for garnish (such as parsley or chives)

Instructions:
1. In a bowl, whisk together the eggs, milk or water, salt, and pepper until well combined.
2. Heat the olive oil in a non-stick skillet over medium heat.
3. Add the minced garlic and sauté for about 30 seconds until fragrant.
4. Add the spinach leaves and cook until they are wilted, about 1-2 minutes.
5. Pour the egg mixture over the spinach in the skillet. Tilt the pan to ensure the eggs are evenly distributed.
6. As the eggs begin to set, gently lift the edges with a spatula and tilt the pan to allow the uncooked eggs to flow to the bottom.
7. When the eggs are almost set but still slightly runny on top, sprinkle the feta cheese over one-half of the omelet.
8. Carefully fold the other half of the omelet over the cheese.
9. Cook for another minute, then slide the omelet onto a plate.
10. Garnish with fresh herbs if desired and serve hot.

Nutritional Facts:
- Calories: 320
- Total Fat: 25g
- Total Carbs: 3g
- Fiber: 1g
- Net Carbs: 2g
- Protein: 20g

Cooking Tip: *For a lighter omelet, use egg whites instead of whole eggs. You can also add other vegetables like tomatoes or bell peppers for added flavor and nutrition. Be careful not to overcook the omelet to keep it fluffy and moist.*

Recipe 3: Avocado Toast with Poached Eggs

Prep Time: 10 mins - Cooking Time: 10 mins - Serves: 2

Ingredients:
2 slices whole-grain bread
1 ripe avocado
2 eggs
1 tablespoon white vinegar (for poaching eggs)
Salt and pepper to taste
Chili flakes to taste
Lemon wedges for serving

Instructions:
1. Toast the whole-grain bread slices to your preferred level of crispiness.
2. Halve the avocado, remove the pit, and scoop out the flesh. Mash the avocado with a fork and season with salt and pepper.
3. Spread the mashed avocado evenly on each slice of toasted bread.
4. To poach the eggs, fill a saucepan with water and add the white vinegar. Bring the water to a gentle simmer.
5. Crack each egg into a small cup or bowl. Gently slide the eggs into the simmering water one at a time. Cook for about 4 minutes, or until the whites are set, but the yolks are still runny.
6. Use a slotted spoon to remove the poached eggs from the water and place them on top of the avocado toast.
7. Sprinkle chili flakes over each egg to taste.
8. Serve the avocado toast with lemon wedges on the side. Squeeze the lemon over the toast just before eating for an added zesty flavor.

Nutritional Facts:
- Calories: 300
- Total Fat: 20g
- Total Carbs: 20g
- Fiber: 7g
- Net Carbs: 13g
- Protein: 12g

Cooking Tip: *For an extra layer of flavor, consider adding chopped herbs like cilantro or parsley to the mashed avocado. If you're new to poaching eggs, swirling the simmering water before adding the eggs can help them hold their shape. For a vegan version, replace the eggs with tofu scramble or seasoned chickpeas.*

Recipe 4: Greek Yogurt Parfait with Mixed Berries

Prep Time: 10 mins - No Cooking - Serves: 2

Ingredients:
2 cups Greek yogurt
1 cup mixed berries (strawberries, blueberries, raspberries, blackberries)
1/2 cup granola
2 tablespoons honey or to taste

Instructions:
1. In two serving glasses or bowls, start by layering 1/4 cup of Greek yogurt at the bottom.
2. Add a layer of mixed berries over the yogurt.
3. Sprinkle a layer of granola on top of the berries.
4. Repeat the layers, starting with the yogurt, then the berries, and finishing with granola, until all ingredients are used.
5. Drizzle honey over the top of each parfait.
6. Serve immediately for a fresh and satisfying breakfast.

Nutritional Facts:
- Calories: 350
- Total Fat: 8g
- Total Carbs: 45g
- Fiber: 4g
- Net Carbs: 41g
- Protein: 25g

Cooking Tip: *For added texture and flavor, mix a pinch of cinnamon or vanilla extract into the Greek yogurt before layering. You can also use different types of granola or add nuts and seeds for extra crunch. For a vegan version, use plant-based yogurt and maple syrup instead of honey.*

Recipe 5: Chia Seed Pudding with Mango

Prep Time: 10 mins - Chill Time: 2 hrs or overnight - Serves: 2

Ingredients:
1/4 cup chia seeds
1 cup almond milk or milk of choice
1 tablespoon honey or maple syrup (optional)
1 ripe mango, diced
2 tablespoons coconut flakes

Instructions:
1. In a bowl, mix together the chia seeds and almond milk. Add honey or maple syrup for sweetness if desired.
2. Stir well to combine and ensure there are no clumps.
3. Cover the bowl and refrigerate for at least 2 hours, or overnight, until the chia seeds have absorbed the liquid and the mixture has a pudding-like consistency.
4. Once the chia pudding is set, give it a good stir to break up any lumps.
5. Divide the chia pudding into two serving bowls or glasses.
6. Top each serving with half of the diced mango and a sprinkle of coconut flakes.
7. Serve chilled as a refreshing and filling breakfast or snack.

Nutritional Facts:
- Calories: 220
- Total Fat: 10g
- Total Carbs: 30g
- Fiber: 10g
- Net Carbs: 20g
- Protein: 5g

Cooking Tip: *For a smoother pudding, blend the chia seed mixture before refrigerating. You can also layer the pudding and mango in a glass for a visually appealing presentation. Experiment with different toppings like berries, nuts, or a drizzle of peanut butter for variety.*

Recipe 6: Quinoa Breakfast Bowl

Prep Time: 5 mins - Cooking Time: 15 mins - Serves: 2

Ingredients:
1 cup cooked quinoa
1/4 cup sliced almonds
1/4 cup dried cranberries
1/2 teaspoon cinnamon
1 cup Greek yogurt
Optional: Honey or maple syrup for drizzling

Instructions:
1. Cook the quinoa according to package instructions. Fluff with a fork and divide it into two serving bowls.
2. Sprinkle the sliced almonds and dried cranberries over the cooked quinoa in each bowl.
3. Dust each serving with a sprinkle of cinnamon for added flavor.
4. Top each bowl with a dollop of Greek yogurt.
5. Optionally, drizzle honey or maple syrup over the top for sweetness.
6. Serve the quinoa breakfast bowls warm for a nourishing and hearty start to your day.

Nutritional Facts:
- Calories: 350
- Total Fat: 10g
- Total Carbs: 50g
- Fiber: 6g
- Net Carbs: 44g
- Protein: 17g

Cooking Tip: *To enhance the flavor of the quinoa, you can cook it in almond milk or coconut milk instead of water. For added crunch and nutrition, sprinkle chia seeds or flaxseeds on top. Feel free to customize it with your favorite fruits, nuts, or seeds. This bowl can also be enjoyed cold, making it a convenient and quick breakfast option.*

Recipe 7: Veggie Breakfast Burrito

Prep Time: 10 mins - Cooking Time: 10 mins - Serves: 2

Ingredients:
4 large eggs
Salt and pepper to taste
1 tablespoon olive oil
1/2 bell pepper, diced
1/2 onion, diced
1/2 cup black beans, drained and rinsed
2 whole wheat tortillas
Optional toppings: shredded cheese, salsa, avocado, sour cream

Instructions:
1. In a bowl, whisk the eggs with salt and pepper.
2. Heat the olive oil in a skillet over medium heat. Add the diced bell pepper and onion, and sauté until they are soft and slightly browned.
3. Pour the whisked eggs into the skillet with the vegetables. Let them sit for a moment without stirring, then gently scramble them until they're just set.
4. Stir in the black beans and cook for an additional minute to warm them through.
5. Warm the whole wheat tortillas in the microwave or on another skillet for a few seconds.
6. Divide the egg and vegetable mixture between the two tortillas, placing it down the center of each tortilla.
7. Add any desired toppings like shredded cheese, salsa, avocado, or sour cream.
8. Roll up each tortilla, tucking in the ends to form a burrito.
9. Serve the veggie breakfast burritos warm.

Nutritional Facts:
- Calories: 350
- Total Fat: 15g
- Total Carbs: 35g
- Fiber: 6g
- Net Carbs: 29g
- Protein: 20g

Cooking Tip: *For a vegan version, use scrambled tofu instead of eggs. You can also add other vegetables like spinach, mushrooms, or zucchini for more variety and nutrition. For added flavor, consider using a flavored tortilla, such as spinach or tomato. If you like it spicy, add some chopped jalapeños or a dash of hot sauce.*

Recipe 8: Overnight Oats with Peanut Butter and Banana

Prep Time: 10 mins - Chill Time: Overnight - Serves: 2

Ingredients:
1 cup rolled oats
1 cup almond milk or milk of choice
2 tablespoons peanut butter
1 ripe banana, sliced
1 tablespoon honey or maple syrup (optional)
1/2 teaspoon vanilla extract
A pinch of salt
Optional toppings: Chia seeds, sliced almonds, or additional banana slices

Instructions:
1. In a medium-sized bowl, combine the rolled oats and almond milk. Stir well.
2. Add the peanut butter, honey, or maple syrup (if using), vanilla extract, and a pinch of salt to the oats. Mix until all ingredients are well incorporated.
3. Gently fold in the sliced banana.
4. Divide the mixture between two jars or containers with lids.
5. Seal the containers and place them in the refrigerator overnight to allow the oats to soak and soften.
6. In the morning, stir the overnight oats and add a little more milk if needed to reach your desired consistency.
7. Top with additional banana slices, chia seeds, or sliced almonds if desired.
8. Serve cold as a convenient and nutritious breakfast option.

Nutritional Facts:
- Calories: 320
- Total Fat: 10g
- Total Carbs: 50g
- Fiber: 7g
- Net Carbs: 43g
- Protein: 10g

Cooking Tip: For a protein boost, add a scoop of your favorite protein powder to the oats before refrigerating. You can also swap the peanut butter with almond butter or any nut butter of your choice. For a gluten-free option, ensure that the oats are certified gluten-free. These overnight oats can be stored in the refrigerator for up to 3 days.

Recipe 9: Smoked Salmon and Cream Cheese Bagel

Prep Time: 5 mins - No Cooking - Serves: 2

Ingredients:
2 whole-grain bagels
4 tablespoons cream cheese
4 ounces smoked salmon
2 tablespoons capers
Thinly sliced red onion
Optional: Fresh dill lemon wedges for garnish

Instructions:
1. Slice the bagels in half and toast them to your preferred level of crispiness.
2. Spread about 1 tablespoon of cream cheese on each bagel half.
3. Arrange the smoked salmon evenly over the cream cheese on each bagel.
4. Sprinkle capers over the smoked salmon.
5. Add a few thin slices of red onion on top for a sharp, crunchy contrast.
6. If desired, garnish with fresh dill and serve with a wedge of lemon on the side.
7. Serve immediately for a classic, flavorful breakfast or brunch.

Nutritional Facts:
- Calories: 370
- Total Fat: 15g
- Total Carbs: 40g
- Fiber: 5g
- Net Carbs: 35g
- Protein: 22g

Cooking Tip*: For added flavor, you can mix some fresh herbs or a pinch of black pepper into the cream cheese before spreading. If you prefer a little heat, add a few slices of fresh jalapeño or a dash of hot sauce. For a lower-carb option, consider using a low-carb or gluten-free bagel.*

Recipe 10: Baked Sweet Potato and Kale Hash

Prep Time: 10 mins - Cooking Time: 30 mins - Serves: 2

Ingredients:
2 large sweet potatoes, peeled and diced
2 tablespoons olive oil, divided
Salt and pepper to taste
1/2 teaspoon paprika
2 cups kale, washed, stems removed, and chopped
2 large eggs
Optional: Crushed red pepper flakes, grated cheese, or fresh herbs for garnish

Instructions:
1. Preheat the oven to 400°F (200°C).
2. Toss the diced sweet potatoes with 1 tablespoon of olive oil, salt, pepper, and paprika. Spread them out in a single layer on a baking sheet.
3. Bake the sweet potatoes for about 20-25 minutes or until tender and lightly browned, stirring halfway through.
4. While the sweet potatoes are baking, heat the remaining tablespoon of olive oil in a large skillet over medium heat.
5. Add the chopped kale and sauté until it's wilted and tender, about 5-7 minutes. Season with salt and pepper to taste.
6. Mix the roasted sweet potatoes into the skillet with the kale and stir to combine. Keep warm.
7. In another skillet, fry the eggs to your desired level of doneness.
8. Divide the sweet potato and kale hash between two plates and top each with a fried egg.
9. Garnish with crushed red pepper flakes, grated cheese, or fresh herbs if desired.
10. Serve immediately for a hearty and nutritious meal.

Nutritional Facts:
- Calories: 380
- Total Fat: 15g
- Total Carbs: 55g
- Fiber: 8g
- Net Carbs: 47g
- Protein: 12g

Cooking Tip: For added protein, you can include diced bacon or sausage in the hash. To add more depth of flavor, consider roasting the sweet potatoes with a mix of cumin and garlic powder. For a vegan option, omit the egg or substitute it with a tofu scramble.

Recipe 11: Blueberry and Walnut Pancakes

Prep Time: 10 mins - Cooking Time: 15 mins - Serves: 4

Ingredients:
1 1/2 cups all-purpose flour
2 tablespoons sugar
1 tablespoon baking powder
1/2 teaspoon salt
1 1/4 cups milk
1 large egg
3 tablespoons unsalted butter, melted
1 teaspoon vanilla extract
1 cup fresh blueberries
1/2 cup walnuts, chopped
Additional butter or oil for cooking
Maple syrup for serving

Instructions:
1. In a large bowl, whisk together the flour, sugar, baking powder, and salt.
2. In another bowl, mix the milk, egg, melted butter, and vanilla extract.
3. Pour the wet ingredients into the dry ingredients and stir until just combined. Be careful not to overmix; some small lumps are okay.
4. Gently fold in the blueberries and chopped walnuts.
5. Heat a non-stick skillet or griddle over medium heat and lightly grease it with butter or oil.
6. Pour 1/4 cup of batter for each pancake onto the skillet. Cook until bubbles form on the surface of the pancakes and the edges start to look set, about 2-3 minutes.
7. Flip the pancakes and cook for another 2-3 minutes until golden brown and cooked through.
8. Serve the pancakes warm with maple syrup on the side.

Nutritional Facts:
- Calories: 350
- Total Fat: 15g
- Total Carbs: 45g
- Fiber: 3g
- Net Carbs: 42g
- Protein: 8g

Cooking Tip: *For lighter pancakes, you can substitute half of the all-purpose flour with whole wheat flour. To keep the pancakes warm while cooking in batches, place them in a preheated oven at 200°F (95°C). If you don't have fresh blueberries, frozen ones can be used without thawing to prevent them from bleeding into the batter.*

Recipe 12: Cottage Cheese and Pineapple Bowl

Prep Time: 5 mins - No Cooking - Serves: 2

Ingredients:
1 cup cottage cheese
1 cup fresh pineapple, cut into chunks
2 tablespoons chia seeds
Optional: Honey or maple syrup for drizzling

Instructions:
1. Divide the cottage cheese evenly between two bowls.
2. Top each bowl with pineapple chunks.
3. Sprinkle 1 tablespoon of chia seeds over each serving.
4. Optionally, drizzle honey or maple syrup over the top for added sweetness.
5. Serve immediately for a refreshing and protein-rich breakfast.

Nutritional Facts:
- Calories: 230
- Total Fat: 7g
- Total Carbs: 25g
- Fiber: 4g
- Net Carbs: 21g
- Protein: 18g

Cooking Tip: *For extra flavor and nutrition, add other fresh fruits like berries or sliced bananas. You can also mix a pinch of cinnamon or vanilla extract into the cottage cheese before serving. For a dairy-free version, use a plant-based cottage cheese substitute. This bowl can be prepared in advance and stored in the refrigerator for a quick and easy breakfast option.*

Chapter 12: Midday Meals - Lunch Favorites

In this chapter, we focus on lunch recipes that are both easy to prepare and delicious. It's all about finding that balance for your midday meals. These recipes cater to preferences and are ideal for giving your body a much-needed energy boost during the day. You'll find an assortment of salads, hearty soups, and light sandwiches that seamlessly fit into a fasting lifestyle.

Recipe 13: Mediterranean Quinoa Salad: Get ready for a burst of colors and healthiness with this salad! It features quinoa, cherry tomatoes, cucumber, olives, and feta cheese, all tossed in a lemon olive oil vinaigrette.

Recipe 14: Roasted Vegetable and Hummus Wrap: Wrap up some deliciousness with this treat! Roasted zucchini, bell peppers, and carrots come together with hummus on a whole wheat tortilla.

Recipe 15: Tomato Basil Soup with Grilled Cheese Croutons: Take comfort in this combination! Indulge in a bowl of comforting tomato soup paired perfectly with grilled cheese croutons for a delightful crunch.

Recipe 16: Asian Chicken Lettuce Wraps: Lighten up your lunchtime with these lettuce wraps! They're filled with stir-fried chicken water chestnuts. Drizzled with an Asian-inspired sauce.

Recipe 17: Avocado and Black Bean Salad: Satisfy your cravings with this salad! Ripe avocados, black beans, corn kernels, and red onion come together in harmony while being tossed in a lime cilantro dressing.

Recipe 18: Tuna and White Bean Salad: Try out a salad that combines tuna, white beans, sliced red onion, and fresh parsley. It's dressed in a vinaigrette that gives it a touch.

Recipe 19: Veggie and Hummus Sandwich: Looking for a sandwich option? Load up on multigrain bread with cucumbers, sprouts, tomatoes, and a creamy hummus spread.

Recipe 20: Sweet Potato and Lentil Soup: Craving something nourishing for lunch? Indulge in a soup made with potatoes, lentils, carrots, and spices. It's perfect for cozying up on days.

Recipe 21: Caprese Pasta Salad: Need an easy yet tasty pasta recipe? Try this one featuring cherry tomatoes, mozzarella balls, and fresh basil, all drizzled with glaze.

Recipe 22: Turkey and Avocado Club Sandwich: Give the club sandwich a twist! Stack your grain bread with turkey slices, avocado slices, crispy bacon strips, lettuce leaves, and tomato slices.

Recipe 23: Spinach and Goat Cheese Salad: Looking for a tangy salad option? Mix baby spinach leaves with creamy goat cheese crumbles and toasted pine nuts. Top it off with a raspberry vinaigrette for that zing.

Recipe 24: Butternut Squash and Chickpea Curry: Warm yourself up with this curry made from butternut squash chunks combined with chickpeas in coconut milk. Serve it over rice for a hearty meal option.

Recipe 13: Mediterranean Quinoa Salad

Prep Time: 15 mins - Cooking Time: 15 mins - Serves: 4

Ingredients:
1 cup quinoa
2 cups water
1 cup cherry tomatoes, halved
1 cucumber, diced
1/2 cup Kalamata olives, pitted and sliced
1/2 cup feta cheese, crumbled
1/4 cup red onion, finely chopped
1/4 cup fresh parsley, chopped
1/4 cup olive oil
Juice of 1 lemon
1 garlic clove, minced
- Salt and pepper to taste

Instructions:
1. Rinse the quinoa under cold water. In a saucepan, bring the quinoa and water to a boil. Reduce the heat, cover, and simmer for about 15 minutes, or until the quinoa is cooked and the water is absorbed.
2. Fluff the cooked quinoa with a fork and let it cool to room temperature.
3. In a large bowl, combine the cooled quinoa, cherry tomatoes, cucumber, Kalamata olives, feta cheese, and red onion.
4. In a small bowl, whisk together the olive oil, lemon juice, minced garlic, salt, and pepper to make the dressing.
5. Pour the dressing over the salad and toss to combine.
6. Garnish with fresh parsley.
7. Adjust the seasoning if necessary and serve the salad at room temperature or chilled.

Nutritional Facts:
- Calories: 320
- Total Fat: 18g
- Total Carbs: 30g
- Fiber: 5g
- Net Carbs: 25g
- Protein: 8g

Cooking Tip: *For an added protein boost, you can include chickpeas or grilled chicken in the salad. To enhance the flavors, let the salad sit for about 30 minutes before serving. You can also add a sprinkle of oregano or mint for extra Mediterranean flair. This salad is versatile and can be adjusted with your favorite veggies or herbs.*

Recipe 14: Roasted Vegetable and Hummus Wrap

Prep Time: 10 mins - Cooking Time: 20 mins - Serves: 2

Ingredients:
1 zucchini, sliced
1 bell pepper, sliced
1 carrot, peeled and sliced
2 tablespoons olive oil
Salt and pepper to taste
1/2 cup hummus
2 whole wheat tortillas
Optional: Baby spinach leaves or arugula

Instructions:
1. Preheat the oven to 400°F (200°C).
2. Place the sliced zucchini, bell pepper, and carrot on a baking sheet. Drizzle with olive oil and season with salt and pepper.
3. Toss the vegetables to coat them evenly and spread them out in a single layer.
4. Roast in the oven for 20 minutes or until the vegetables are tender and lightly browned, turning halfway through.
5. Warm the whole wheat tortillas in the microwave or on a skillet for a few seconds.
6. Spread a layer of hummus on each tortilla.
7. Evenly distribute the roasted vegetables over the hummus.
8. If using, add a layer of baby spinach or arugula.
9. Roll up the tortillas tightly to enclose the filling.
10. Serve immediately or wrap them up for a convenient and nutritious on-the-go meal.

Nutritional Facts:
- Calories: 320
- Total Fat: 15g
- Total Carbs: 40g
- Fiber: 7g
- Net Carbs: 33g
- Protein: 10g

Cooking Tip: *For added flavor, you can sprinkle your favorite herbs or spices, such as rosemary, thyme, or paprika, on the vegetables before roasting. For a gluten-free option, use gluten-free tortillas. You can also add grilled chicken or tofu for a protein boost. The wrap can be served warm or cold, making it a versatile meal option.*

Recipe 15: Tomato Basil Soup with Grilled Cheese Croutons

Prep Time: 15 mins - Cooking Time: 30 mins - Serves: 4

Ingredients:
For the Tomato Basil Soup:
2 tablespoons olive oil
1 onion, finely chopped
2 garlic cloves, minced
1 can (28 ounces) crushed tomatoes
2 cups vegetable broth
1/4 cup fresh basil leaves, chopped
Salt and pepper to taste
1/2 cup heavy cream or coconut milk (optional)

For the Grilled Cheese Croutons:
- 4 slices whole-grain bread
- 4 slices cheddar cheese
- 2 tablespoons butter

Instructions:
1. In a large pot, heat the olive oil over medium heat. Add the chopped onion and minced garlic, and sauté until the onion is translucent.
2. Stir in the crushed tomatoes and vegetable broth. Bring to a simmer.
3. Add the chopped basil, salt, and pepper. Let the soup simmer for about 20 minutes, stirring occasionally.
4. While the soup is simmering, make the grilled cheese sandwiches. Butter one side of each bread slice. Place a slice of cheese between two slices of bread, with the buttered sides facing outward.
5. Heat a skillet over medium heat. Cook the sandwiches for about 2-3 minutes on each side, until golden brown and the cheese is melted.
6. Remove the grilled cheese sandwiches from the skillet and let them cool slightly. Cut into small, bite-sized squares to create croutons.
7. Optional: For a creamier soup, stir in the heavy cream or coconut milk after the soup has finished simmering.
8. Serve the tomato basil soup hot, topped with the grilled cheese croutons.

Nutritional Facts:
- Calories: 380
- Total Fat: 22g
- Total Carbs: 35g
- Fiber: 5g
- Net Carbs: 30g
- Protein: 12g

Cooking Tip: *For a vegan version, use vegan cheese slices and a dairy-free butter alternative for the croutons. Opt for coconut milk in the soup. You can also add a carrot or celery stalk with the onion for extra flavor.*

Recipe 16: Asian Chicken Lettuce Wraps

Prep Time: 15 mins - Cooking Time: 10 mins - Serves: 4

Ingredients:
1 pound ground chicken
1 tablespoon vegetable oil
1 large onion, diced
2 garlic cloves, minced
1 tablespoon fresh ginger, grated
1 can (8 ounces) water chestnuts, drained and finely chopped
1/4 cup soy sauce
2 tablespoons hoisin sauce
1 tablespoon rice vinegar
1 teaspoon sesame oil
1 head of lettuce, leaves separated (Bibb or iceberg)
Optional toppings: Sliced green onions, sesame seeds, cilantro, or crushed peanuts

Instructions:
1. Heat the vegetable oil in a skillet over medium-high heat. Add the ground chicken and cook, breaking it apart with a spatula, until browned and cooked through.
2. Add the diced onion, minced garlic, and grated ginger to the skillet with the chicken. Cook for a few minutes until the onion softens.
3. Stir in the chopped water chestnuts, soy sauce, hoisin sauce, rice vinegar, and sesame oil. Cook for another 2-3 minutes, stirring frequently, until everything is well combined and heated through.
4. Carefully separate the lettuce leaves, wash them, and pat them dry.
5. To assemble the wraps, spoon a generous amount of the chicken mixture into the center of each lettuce leaf.
6. Add any optional toppings like sliced green onions, sesame seeds, cilantro, or crushed peanuts.
7. Serve the lettuce wraps immediately, allowing diners to wrap and eat them with their hands.

Nutritional Facts:
- Calories: 250
- Total Fat: 12g
- Total Carbs: 10g
- Fiber: 2g
- Net Carbs: 8g
- Protein: 25g

Cooking Tip*: For a spicier kick, add a tablespoon of Sriracha or chili garlic sauce to the chicken mixture. The lettuce wraps can also be served with a side of extra hoisin sauce or sweet chili sauce for dipping. If you're looking for a vegetarian option, substitute the chicken with tofu or tempeh.*

Recipe 17: Avocado and Black Bean Salad

Prep Time: 15 mins - No Cooking - Serves: 4

Ingredients:
2 ripe avocados, diced
1 can (15 ounces) black beans, drained and rinsed
1 cup corn kernels, fresh, canned, or thawed from frozen
1/2 red onion, finely chopped
1/4 cup fresh cilantro, chopped
Juice of 2 limes
2 tablespoons olive oil
Salt and pepper to taste
Optional: Cherry tomatoes, halved, or diced bell pepper for added color

Instructions:
1. In a large bowl, gently toss the diced avocados, black beans, corn, and chopped red onion.
2. In a small bowl, whisk together the lime juice, olive oil, salt, and pepper to create the dressing.
3. Pour the dressing over the salad and gently toss to coat all the ingredients.
4. Add the chopped cilantro and give the salad a final toss.
5. If using, mix in cherry tomatoes or diced bell pepper.
6. Taste and adjust the seasoning if necessary.
7. Serve the avocado and black bean salad chilled or at room temperature.

Nutritional Facts:
- Calories: 290
- Total Fat: 15g
- Total Carbs: 35g
- Fiber: 12g
- Net Carbs: 23g
- Protein: 9g

Cooking Tip: *For an extra protein boost, add grilled chicken or shrimp. You can also include a sprinkle of cumin or chili powder for a warm, smoky flavor. If you're making this salad ahead of time, add the avocado just before serving to prevent browning. This salad pairs well with tortilla chips or as a filling for tacos or burritos.*

Recipe 18: Tuna and White Bean Salad

Prep Time: 10 mins - No Cooking - Serves: 4

Ingredients:
2 cans (each 5 ounces) of tuna in water, drained and flaked
1 can (15 ounces) white beans (such as cannellini or Great Northern), drained and rinsed
1/2 red onion, thinly sliced
1/4 cup fresh parsley, chopped
3 tablespoons olive oil
2 tablespoons red wine vinegar
1 garlic clove, minced
Salt and pepper to taste
Optional: Cherry tomatoes, halved, or cucumber slices

Instructions:
1. In a large bowl, combine the flaked tuna and white beans.
2. Add the sliced red onion and chopped parsley to the bowl.
3. In a small bowl, whisk together the olive oil, red wine vinegar, minced garlic, salt, and pepper to create the vinaigrette.
4. Pour the vinaigrette over the tuna and bean mixture. Toss gently to ensure everything is evenly coated.
5. If using, add cherry tomatoes or cucumber slices to the salad.
6. Taste and adjust the seasoning if necessary.
7. Serve the salad chilled or at room temperature.

Nutritional Facts:
- Calories: 240
- Total Fat: 10g
- Total Carbs: 20g
- Fiber: 5g
- Net Carbs: 15g
- Protein: 20g

Cooking Tip: *For added crunch, include diced bell pepper or celery. A squeeze of fresh lemon juice can be added for extra zing. This salad can be served on its own, over a bed of greens, or as a filling for a wrap or sandwich. If preparing in advance, add the dressing just before serving to keep the salad fresh.*

Recipe 19: Veggie and Hummus Sandwich

Prep Time: 10 mins - No Cooking - Serves: 2

Ingredients:
4 slices multigrain bread
1/2 cup hummus
1 cucumber, thinly sliced
1 cup alfalfa sprouts or mixed sprouts
1 large tomato, thinly sliced
Salt and pepper to taste
Optional: Avocado slices, red onion rings, or spinach leaves

Instructions:
1. Lightly toast the multigrain bread slices if desired.
2. Spread a generous layer of hummus on one side of each bread slice.
3. On two of the bread slices, layer the cucumber slices, sprouts, and tomato slices. Season with salt and pepper.
4. If using, add avocado slices, red onion rings, or spinach leaves for additional flavor and nutrients.
5. Top with the remaining bread slices, hummus side down, to complete the sandwiches.
6. Cut the sandwiches in half and serve immediately.

Nutritional Facts:
- Calories: 330
- Total Fat: 9g
- Total Carbs: 49g
- Fiber: 13g
- Net Carbs: 36g
- Protein: 12g

Cooking Tip: *For a gluten-free option, use gluten-free bread. You can also add a drizzle of olive oil or balsamic vinegar for extra flavor. This sandwich is versatile and can be customized with your favorite vegetables or additions like sliced bell peppers or shredded carrots. For a heartier meal, add a slice of cheese or grilled chicken.*

Recipe 20: Sweet Potato and Lentil Soup

Prep Time: 15 mins - Cooking Time: 30 mins - Serves: 4

Ingredients:
1 tablespoon olive oil
1 onion, chopped
2 garlic cloves, minced
1 large sweet potato, peeled and diced
2 carrots, peeled and diced
1 cup dried lentils, rinsed
4 cups vegetable broth
1 teaspoon ground cumin
1/2 teaspoon ground coriander
1/2 teaspoon paprika
Salt and pepper to taste
Optional: Chopped fresh parsley or cilantro for garnish

Instructions:
1. Heat the olive oil in a large pot over medium heat. Add the chopped onion and minced garlic, and sauté until the onion is translucent.
2. Add the diced sweet potato and carrots to the pot. Cook for about 5 minutes, stirring occasionally.
3. Stir in the lentils, vegetable broth, cumin, coriander, and paprika. Bring the mixture to a boil.
4. Reduce the heat to low, cover the pot, and simmer for about 20-25 minutes or until the lentils and vegetables are tender.
5. Season the soup with salt and pepper to taste.
6. Optionally, use an immersion blender to partially puree the soup for a creamier texture, or leave it as is for a chunkier soup.
7. Serve the soup hot, garnished with chopped parsley or cilantro if desired.

Nutritional Facts:
- Calories: 280
- Total Fat: 4g
- Total Carbs: 48g
- Fiber: 19g
- Net Carbs: 29g
- Protein: 14g

Cooking Tip: *For a heartier soup, you can add chopped kale or spinach in the last few minutes of cooking. A squeeze of lemon juice added before serving can enhance the flavors. This soup can be stored in the refrigerator for up to 3 days or frozen for longer storage.*

Recipe 21: Caprese Pasta Salad

Prep Time: 15 mins - Cooking Time: 10 mins - Serves: 4

Ingredients:

8 ounces of pasta (such as penne, rotini, or farfalle)
1 1/2 cups cherry tomatoes, halved
1 cup mozzarella balls (bocconcini), halved
1/4 cup fresh basil leaves, torn or chopped
1/4 cup balsamic glaze
2 tablespoons olive oil
Salt and pepper to taste
Optional: Crushed red pepper flakes for a spicy kick

Instructions:

1. Cook the pasta according to package instructions until al dente. Drain and rinse under cold water to cool.
2. In a large bowl, combine the cooled pasta, cherry tomatoes, mozzarella balls, and fresh basil.
3. Drizzle the olive oil and balsamic glaze over the salad. Toss gently to coat all the ingredients evenly.
4. Season the salad with salt, pepper, and crushed red pepper flakes if using. Toss again.
5. Let the pasta salad chill in the refrigerator for at least 30 minutes before serving to allow the flavors to meld.
6. Serve the Caprese pasta salad as a refreshing side dish or light main course.

Nutritional Facts:

- Calories: 350
- Total Fat: 14g
- Total Carbs: 45g
- Fiber: 2g
- Net Carbs: 43g
- Protein: 12g

***Cooking Tip:** For a healthier version, use whole wheat or gluten-free pasta. You can also add extra vegetables like spinach, arugula, or diced cucumber for more nutrition and flavor. The balsamic glaze can be substituted with a mixture of balsamic vinegar and a little honey or maple syrup. For added protein, consider adding grilled chicken or shrimp.*

Recipe 22: Turkey and Avocado Club Sandwich

Prep Time: 10 mins - No Cooking - Serves: 2

Ingredients:
4 slices whole grain bread
4 slices cooked turkey breast
4 slices of cooked bacon
1 ripe avocado, sliced
4 lettuce leaves
1 tomato, sliced
2 tablespoons mayonnaise or Greek yogurt
Salt and pepper to taste
Optional: Mustard or honey mustard

Instructions:
1. Toast the whole grain bread slices to your desired level of crispness.
2. Spread mayonnaise (or Greek yogurt) on one side of each bread slice. If using, add mustard as well.
3. On two of the bread slices, layer the cooked turkey breast slices.
4. Add the cooked bacon on top of the turkey.
5. Place the lettuce leaves and tomato slices over the bacon. Season with salt and pepper.
6. Add the avocado slices on top of the tomatoes.
7. Cover with the remaining bread slices, mayonnaise side down.
8. Carefully cut each sandwich in half or into quarters and secure it with toothpicks if needed.
9. Serve the turkey and avocado club sandwiches immediately.

Nutritional Facts:
- Calories: 450
- Total Fat: 20g
- Total Carbs: 40g
- Fiber: 8g
- Net Carbs: 32g
- Protein: 30g

Cooking Tip: *For a lighter version, use a low-fat mayonnaise or Greek yogurt. You can also add additional vegetables like cucumber or sprouts for extra crunch and nutrition. For a gluten-free option, use gluten-free bread. This sandwich is versatile and can be customized to include your favorite sandwich fillings.*

Recipe 23: Spinach and Goat Cheese Salad

Prep Time: 10 mins - No Cooking - Serves: 4

Ingredients:
6 cups baby spinach leaves, washed and dried
1/2 cup goat cheese, crumbled
1/4 cup pine nuts, toasted
1/2 cup fresh raspberries (optional for the vinaigrette and garnish)
For the Raspberry Vinaigrette:
1/4 cup raspberry vinegar
1/2 cup olive oil
1 tablespoon honey or maple syrup
Salt and pepper to taste
Optional add-ins: Sliced red onion, avocado slices, or dried cranberries

Instructions:
1. In a dry skillet over medium heat, lightly toast the pine nuts until golden brown, stirring frequently to prevent burning. Set aside to cool.
2. In a large salad bowl, combine the baby spinach leaves with the crumbled goat cheese and toasted pine nuts.
3. To prepare the raspberry vinaigrette, whisk together the raspberry vinegar, olive oil, and honey or maple syrup in a small bowl. Season with salt and pepper.
4. Drizzle the vinaigrette over the salad and toss gently to combine all the ingredients.
5. If using, add fresh raspberries, sliced red onion, avocado slices, or dried cranberries to the salad for extra flavor and texture.
6. Serve the spinach and goat cheese salad immediately, garnished with additional raspberries if desired.

Nutritional Facts:
- Calories: 290
- Total Fat: 24g
- Total Carbs: 14g
- Fiber: 3g
- Net Carbs: 11g
- Protein: 7g

Cooking Tip: *For a more substantial salad, you can add grilled chicken or shrimp. The raspberry vinaigrette can be made in advance and stored in the refrigerator. Feel free to adjust the ingredients of the vinaigrette to suit your taste, such as adding more honey for sweetness or more vinegar for acidity. This salad is perfect as a light lunch or as a side dish for a larger meal.*

Recipe 24: Butternut Squash and Chickpea Curry

Prep Time: 15 mins - Cooking Time: 30 mins - Serves: 4

Ingredients:
1 tablespoon vegetable oil
1 onion, diced
2 garlic cloves, minced
1 tablespoon grated ginger
1 butternut squash, peeled and cubed (about 4 cups)
1 can (15 ounces) chickpeas, drained and rinsed
1 can (14 ounces) coconut milk
2 tablespoons curry powder
1 teaspoon ground cumin
1/2 teaspoon ground turmeric
Salt and pepper to taste
2 cups cooked brown rice
Optional: Fresh cilantro for garnish, lime wedges for serving

Instructions:
1. Heat the vegetable oil in a large pot over medium heat. Add the diced onion and cook until soft and translucent.
2. Add the minced garlic and grated ginger, cooking for another minute until fragrant.
3. Stir in the curry powder, cumin, and turmeric until the onions are well coated.
4. Add the cubed butternut squash and chickpeas to the pot. Stir to combine with the spices.
5. Pour in the coconut milk and bring the mixture to a simmer. Reduce the heat, cover, and let it cook for about 20 minutes or until the butternut squash is tender.
6. Season the curry with salt and pepper to taste.
7. Serve the curry over cooked brown rice, garnished with fresh cilantro and lime wedges on the side.

Nutritional Facts:
- Calories: 450
- Total Fat: 18g
- Total Carbs: 65g
- Fiber: 10g
- Net Carbs: 55g
- Protein: 12g

Cooking Tip: *For added depth of flavor, consider adding a teaspoon of garam masala. You can also include vegetables like spinach or bell peppers for more nutrition and color. If you prefer a spicier curry, add some red chili flakes or a diced chili pepper. This curry can be stored in the refrigerator for up to 3 days and is ideal for meal prep.*

Chapter 13: The Heart of Dining - Main Course Creations

In this chapter, we explore the essence of meal planning by offering a variety of course recipes. These recipes encompass a range of traditions and cater to different dietary preferences, including options for vegetarians, vegans, and those who enjoy meat. Not are these dishes nutritious. They also boast delicious flavors that guarantee a satisfying dining experience while adhering to the principles of intermittent fasting.

Recipe 25: Grilled Chicken with Lemon and Herbs: Tender chicken breasts marinated in lemon juice, garlic, and aromatic herbs. They are then grilled to perfection, resulting in a delicious meal.

Recipe 26: Vegan Mushroom Stroganoff: A substantial vegan adaptation of the stroganoff recipe. This version features mushrooms complemented by a cashew-based sauce served over wheat pasta.

Recipe 27: Baked Salmon with Dill Sauce: Delicate salmon fillets expertly baked in the oven. Topped with a dill-infused yogurt sauce. Served alongside asparagus for a combination.

Recipe 28: Thai Green Curry with Tofu: A fiery Thai curry bursting with flavors. This dish showcases tofu along with bell peppers, and broccoli served over jasmine rice.

Recipe 29: Chickpea and Vegetable Tagine: An aromatic and spiced stew featuring chickpeas, sweet potatoes, carrots, and an enticing blend of seasonings. Served alongside couscous for a taste experience.

Here are some delicious recipes for you to try:

Recipe 30: Beef and Broccoli Stir Fry: Experience the blend of tender beef slices and broccoli combined in a mouthwatering marinade made with soy sauce and ginger.

Recipe 31: Cauliflower and Chickpea Masala: Indulge in the flavors of India with this dish featuring cauliflower and chickpeas immersed in a rich tomato-based masala sauce.

Recipe 32: Shrimp and Zucchini Noodles: Treat yourself to a nutritious meal comprising sautéed shrimp paired with spiralized zucchini noodles, all tossed in a garlic lemon sauce.

Recipe 33: Stuffed Bell Peppers: Delight your taste buds with bell peppers filled with a mixture of ground turkey, quinoa, tomatoes, and spices. Bake them until they turn tender for a dining experience.

Recipe 34: Eggplant Parmesan: Enjoy the goodness of slices of eggplant layered with marinara sauce and mozzarella cheese. It's a treat!

Recipe 35: Pork Tenderloin with Apple Cider Glaze: Prepare yourself for a succulent pork tenderloin roasted to perfection and coated in a tangy apple cider glaze. Served alongside root vegetables for a meal.

Recipe 36: Vegetarian Black Bean Enchiladas: Savor these hearty enchiladas stuffed with beans, corn, and cheese. Smothered generously in enchilada sauce before being baked to bubbly perfection.

Recipe 25: Grilled Lemon Herb Chicken

Prep Time: 20 mins (including marinating time) - Cooking Time: 10 mins - Serves: 4

Ingredients:
4 boneless, skinless chicken breasts
1/4 cup olive oil
Juice of 2 lemons
3 garlic cloves, minced
1 tablespoon fresh rosemary, chopped
1 tablespoon fresh thyme, chopped
1 teaspoon dried oregano
Salt and pepper to taste
Lemon slices and additional herbs for garnish

Instructions:

1. In a bowl, whisk together the olive oil, lemon juice, minced garlic, chopped rosemary, thyme, oregano, salt, and pepper to create the marinade.
2. Place the chicken breasts in a resealable plastic bag or shallow dish. Pour the marinade over the chicken, ensuring each piece is well coated.
3. Marinate the chicken in the refrigerator for at least 15 minutes or up to 2 hours for more flavor.
4. Preheat the grill to medium-high heat.
5. Remove the chicken from the marinade and grill for about 5 minutes on each side or until the chicken is thoroughly cooked and has nice grill marks.
6. Let the chicken rest for a few minutes before serving.
7. Serve the grilled chicken with lemon slices and a sprinkle of fresh herbs.

Nutritional Facts:
- Calories: 220
- Total Fat: 10g
- Total Carbs: 1g
- Fiber: 0g
- Net Carbs: 1g
- Protein: 30g

***Cooking Tip:** To ensure the chicken cooks evenly, pound the breasts to an even thickness before marinating. You can also cut slits in the chicken to help it absorb more flavor. If you don't have a grill, this recipe can be adapted for a grill pan or skillet. For a complete meal, serve the chicken with a side of grilled vegetables or a fresh salad.*

Recipe 26: Vegan Mushroom Stroganoff

Prep Time: 15 mins - Cooking Time: 20 mins - Serves: 4

Ingredients:
1 cup raw cashews, soaked for 2 hours and drained
2 tablespoons olive oil
1 onion, finely chopped
3 garlic cloves, minced
1 pound of sliced mushrooms (such as cremini or portobello)
2 tablespoons soy sauce or tamari
1 teaspoon smoked paprika
1/2 teaspoon ground black pepper
2 cups vegetable broth
1 tablespoon cornstarch dissolved in 2 tablespoons water
8 ounces whole wheat pasta
Chopped fresh parsley for garnish
Optional: Nutritional yeast for a cheesy flavor

Instructions:
1. Cook the whole wheat pasta according to package instructions until al dente. Drain and set aside.
2. In a blender, combine the soaked and drained cashews with 1 cup of vegetable broth. Blend until smooth and creamy. Set aside.
3. In a large skillet, heat the olive oil over medium heat. Add the onion and garlic, and sauté until the onion is translucent.
4. Add the sliced mushrooms to the skillet and cook until they are browned and their moisture has evaporated.
5. Stir in the soy sauce or tamari, smoked paprika, and ground black pepper.
6. Add the remaining 1 cup of vegetable broth to the skillet and bring to a simmer.
7. Stir in the cornstarch mixture and the blended cashew cream. Cook, stirring continuously, until the sauce thickens.
8. Reduce the heat to low and let the stroganoff simmer for a few more minutes to blend the flavors.
9. Serve the mushroom stroganoff over the cooked pasta, garnished with chopped parsley.
10. Optionally, sprinkle nutritional yeast over the top for added flavor.

Nutritional Facts:
- Calories: 410
- Total Fat: 20g
- Total Carbs: 47g
- Fiber: 8g
- Net Carbs: 39g
- Protein: 15g

***Cooking Tip:** If you're short on time, you can use a high-powered blender to make the cashew cream without soaking the cashews. For a gluten-free version, use gluten-free pasta. The mushroom stroganoff can also be served over rice, quinoa, or mashed potatoes. Feel free to add other vegetables, like spinach or peas, to the stroganoff for added nutrition and color.*

Recipe 27: Baked Salmon with Dill Sauce

Prep Time: 10 mins - Cooking Time: 15 mins - Serves: 4

Ingredients:
For the Salmon:
4 salmon fillets (about 6 ounces each)
2 tablespoons olive oil
Salt and pepper to taste
1 lemon, sliced for garnish

For the Dill Sauce:
1 cup Greek yogurt
2 tablespoons fresh dill, chopped
1 tablespoon lemon juice
1 garlic clove, minced
Salt and pepper to taste

For the Asparagus:
1 pound asparagus, ends trimmed
1 tablespoon olive oil
Salt and pepper to taste

Instructions:
1. Preheat the oven to 400°F (200°C). Line a baking sheet with parchment paper.
2. Place the salmon fillets on the baking sheet. Drizzle with olive oil and season with salt and pepper.
3. Bake the salmon in the preheated oven for 12-15 minutes or until the fish flakes easily with a fork.
4. While the salmon is baking, make the dill sauce. In a small bowl, mix together the Greek yogurt, chopped dill, lemon juice, minced garlic, salt, and pepper.
5. For the asparagus, toss the trimmed asparagus with olive oil, salt, and pepper. Steam or sauté until tender, about 3-5 minutes.
6. Serve the baked salmon with a generous dollop of dill sauce and a side of steamed asparagus. Garnish with lemon slices.

Nutritional Facts:
- Calories: 380
- Total Fat: 20g
- Total Carbs: 5g
- Fiber: 2g
- Net Carbs: 3g
- Protein: 40g

Cooking Tip: *For added flavor, marinate the salmon in a mixture of lemon juice, olive oil, and herbs for at least 30 minutes before baking. You can also grill the salmon for a smoky flavor. The dill sauce can be made ahead of time and stored in the refrigerator. Feel free to add capers or chopped cucumber to the sauce for extra texture and flavor.*

Recipe 28: Thai Green Curry with Tofu

Prep Time: 15 mins - Cooking Time: 20 mins - Serves: 4

Ingredients:
14 ounces of firm tofu, pressed and cut into cubes
2 tablespoons vegetable oil
1 onion, sliced
2 bell peppers (one red, one green), sliced
1 head of broccoli, cut into florets
3 tablespoons Thai green curry paste
1 can (14 ounces) coconut milk
1 tablespoon soy sauce or tamari
1 tablespoon brown sugar or maple syrup
1/2 cup fresh basil leaves
2 cups jasmine rice, cooked according to package instructions

Instructions:
1. Heat 1 tablespoon of vegetable oil in a large skillet or wok over medium heat. Add the tofu cubes and fry until all sides are golden brown. Remove from the skillet and set aside.
2. In the same skillet, heat the remaining 1 tablespoon of oil. Add the sliced onion and bell peppers, and sauté until they start to soften.
3. Add the broccoli florets and continue to cook for a few more minutes until they're bright green and slightly tender.
4. Stir in the Thai green curry paste, ensuring the vegetables are well coated.
5. Pour in the coconut milk, soy sauce or tamari, and brown sugar or maple syrup. Stir well to combine.
6. Bring the curry to a simmer, then add the fried tofu back into the skillet. Cook for another 5 minutes, allowing the flavors to meld together.
7. Just before serving, stir in the fresh basil leaves.
8. Serve the Thai green curry over cooked jasmine rice.

Nutritional Facts:
- Calories: 510
- Total Fat: 24g
- Total Carbs: 60g
- Fiber: 4g
- Net Carbs: 56g
- Protein: 18g

Cooking Tip: *For a more authentic flavor, add Thai ingredients like kaffir lime leaves, lemongrass, or galangal if available. You can also add other vegetables like snap peas, carrots, or baby corn. For a spicier curry, include some Thai green chilies. If you're not vegan or vegetarian, you can substitute the tofu with chicken or shrimp.*

Recipe 29: Moroccan Chickpea and Vegetable Tagine

Prep Time: 15 mins - Cooking Time: 40 mins - Serves: 4

Ingredients:
2 tablespoons olive oil
1 large onion, chopped
3 garlic cloves, minced
1 teaspoon ground cumin
1 teaspoon ground coriander
1/2 teaspoon ground cinnamon
1/2 teaspoon paprika
1/4 teaspoon ground ginger
1 can (15 ounces) chickpeas, drained and rinsed
2 sweet potatoes, peeled and cubed
2 large carrots, peeled and sliced
1 can (14 ounces) diced tomatoes with juice
3 cups vegetable broth
Salt and pepper to taste
1/2 cup dried apricots, chopped
2 cups couscous, cooked according to package instructions
Fresh cilantro or parsley for garnish

Instructions:
1. Heat the olive oil in a large pot or tagine over medium heat. Add the chopped onion and sauté until translucent.
2. Add the minced garlic, cumin, coriander, cinnamon, paprika, and ginger. Cook for another minute until fragrant.
3. Stir in the chickpeas, sweet potatoes, and carrots. Cook for a few minutes, stirring occasionally.
4. Add the diced tomatoes with their juice and the vegetable broth. Season with salt and pepper.
5. Bring the mixture to a simmer, then reduce the heat, cover, and cook for about 30 minutes or until the vegetables are tender.
6. Stir in the chopped dried apricots and cook for an additional 10 minutes.
7. Serve the Moroccan chickpea and vegetable tagine over cooked couscous, garnished with fresh cilantro or parsley.

Nutritional Facts:
- Calories: 480
- Total Fat: 8g
- Total Carbs: 85g
- Fiber: 15g
- Net Carbs: 70g
- Protein: 15g

Cooking Tip: For a richer flavor, you can add a pinch of saffron or a splash of orange juice to the tagine. This dish can be customized with additional vegetables like zucchini, bell peppers, or turnips. For a non-vegetarian version, you can add chicken or lamb. Leftover tagine can be stored in the refrigerator for up to 3 days and reheats well.

Recipe 30: Beef and Broccoli Stir-Fry

Prep Time: 15 mins (plus marinating time) - Cooking Time: 10 mins - Serves: 4

Ingredients:
For the Marinade:
1/2 cup soy sauce
2 tablespoons brown sugar
1 tablespoon sesame oil
2 garlic cloves, minced
1 tablespoon fresh ginger, grated

For the Stir-Fry:
1 pound beef (such as flank steak or sirloin), thinly sliced against the grain
3 tablespoons vegetable oil, divided
4 cups broccoli florets
1 onion, sliced
1/4 cup water or beef broth
1 tablespoon cornstarch mixed with 2 tablespoons water (slurry)
Optional: Sesame seeds and sliced green onions for garnish

Instructions:
1. In a bowl, whisk together the soy sauce, brown sugar, sesame oil, minced garlic, and grated ginger to make the marinade.
2. Place the thinly sliced beef in the marinade and let it sit in the refrigerator for at least 30 minutes or up to 2 hours.
3. Heat 2 tablespoons of vegetable oil in a large skillet or wok over high heat. Add the marinated beef (reserve the marinade) and stir-fry until browned and cooked through. Remove the beef from the skillet and set aside.
4. In the same skillet, add the remaining 1 tablespoon of oil. Add the broccoli and onion, and stir-fry for a few minutes until the vegetables are tender-crisp.
5. Add the reserved marinade and water or beef broth to the skillet. Bring to a simmer.
6. Stir in the cornstarch slurry and cook until the sauce thickens.
7. Return the cooked beef to the skillet and toss everything together until the beef and broccoli are well coated with the sauce.
8. Serve the beef and broccoli stir-fry hot, garnished with sesame seeds and sliced green onions if desired.

Nutritional Facts:
- Calories: 320
- Total Fat: 15g
- Total Carbs: 15g
- Fiber: 2g
- Net Carbs: 13g
- Protein: 30g

Cooking Tip: For extra flavor, marinate the beef overnight. If you prefer a spicier dish, add red pepper flakes to the marinade.

Recipe 31: Cauliflower and Chickpea Masala

Prep Time: 15 mins - Cooking Time: 30 mins - Serves: 4

Ingredients:
- 1 head cauliflower, cut into florets
- 1 can (15 ounces) chickpeas, drained and rinsed
- 2 tablespoons vegetable oil, divided
- Salt and pepper to taste
- 1 onion, finely chopped
- 2 garlic cloves, minced
- 1 tablespoon fresh ginger, grated
- 2 teaspoons garam masala
- 1 teaspoon ground cumin
- 1/2 teaspoon turmeric
- 1/4 teaspoon cayenne pepper (optional, for heat)
- 1 can (14 ounces) crushed tomatoes
- 1 cup coconut milk or cream
- Fresh cilantro for garnish
- Cooked rice or naan bread for serving

Instructions:
1. Preheat the oven to 400°F (200°C). Toss the cauliflower florets and chickpeas with 1 tablespoon of vegetable oil, salt, and pepper. Spread them on a baking sheet and roast for 20 minutes or until the cauliflower is tender and golden.
2. While the cauliflower and chickpeas are roasting, heat the remaining 1 tablespoon of oil in a large skillet over medium heat. Add the chopped onion and cook until soft.
3. Add the minced garlic, grated ginger, garam masala, cumin, turmeric, and cayenne pepper. Cook for 1-2 minutes until fragrant.
4. Stir in the crushed tomatoes and bring the mixture to a simmer.
5. Add the coconut milk or cream to the skillet and continue to simmer the sauce for about 10 minutes or until it thickens slightly.
6. Once the cauliflower and chickpeas are roasted, add them to the skillet with the masala sauce. Toss to coat everything evenly.
7. Garnish with fresh cilantro and serve the cauliflower and chickpea masala with cooked rice or warm naan bread.

Nutritional Facts:
- Calories: 380
- Total Fat: 20g
- Total Carbs: 40g
- Fiber: 10g
- Net Carbs: 30g
- Protein: 13g

Cooking Tip: *For added depth of flavor, you can include a pinch of ground cinnamon or cardamom in the masala sauce.*

Recipe 32: Shrimp and Zucchini Noodles

Prep Time: 15 mins - Cooking Time: 10 mins - Serves: 4

Ingredients:
1 pound large shrimp, peeled and deveined
4 medium zucchinis, spiralized into noodles
2 tablespoons olive oil, divided
3 garlic cloves, minced
Juice and zest of 1 lemon
Salt and pepper to taste
Red pepper flakes to taste (optional)
Fresh parsley, chopped for garnish
Grated Parmesan cheese for serving (optional)

Instructions:
1. Pat the shrimp dry with paper towels and season with salt and pepper.
2. Heat 1 tablespoon of olive oil in a large skillet over medium-high heat. Add the shrimp and cook for 1-2 minutes on each side or until they are pink and opaque. Remove the shrimp from the skillet and set aside.
3. In the same skillet, add the remaining 1 tablespoon of olive oil. Sauté the minced garlic for about 1 minute until fragrant.
4. Add the spiralized zucchini noodles to the skillet. Toss them with the garlic and cook for 2-3 minutes until just tender.
5. Return the shrimp to the skillet with the zucchini noodles. Add the lemon juice, lemon zest, and red pepper flakes (if using). Toss everything together and heat through.
6. Season with additional salt and pepper to taste.
7. Serve the shrimp and zucchini noodles garnished with chopped parsley and grated Parmesan cheese, if desired.

Nutritional Facts:
- Calories: 220
- Total Fat: 9g
- Total Carbs: 8g
- Fiber: 2g
- Net Carbs: 6g
- Protein: 28g

Cooking Tip: *To prevent the zucchini noodles from becoming too watery, don't overcook them; they should be al dente. For added flavor, you can include a splash of white wine or chicken broth when cooking the shrimp. This dish is versatile and can be customized with other herbs like basil or dill. For a vegetarian option, replace the shrimp with tofu or extra vegetables.*

Recipe 33: Stuffed Bell Peppers

Prep Time: 20 mins - Cooking Time: 30 mins - Serves: 4

Ingredients:
4 bell peppers, tops cut off and seeds removed
1 tablespoon olive oil
1 pound ground turkey
1 onion, chopped
2 garlic cloves, minced
1 cup cooked quinoa
1 can (14 ounces) diced tomatoes, drained
1 teaspoon ground cumin
1 teaspoon paprika
1/2 teaspoon dried oregano
Salt and pepper to taste
1/2 cup shredded cheese (such as cheddar or mozzarella), optional
Fresh parsley, chopped for garnish

Instructions:
1. Preheat the oven to 375°F (190°C).
2. Heat the olive oil in a skillet over medium heat. Add the ground turkey and cook until browned, breaking it apart with a spatula.
3. Add the chopped onion and minced garlic to the skillet with the turkey. Cook until the onion is soft.
4. Stir in the cooked quinoa, diced tomatoes, cumin, paprika, oregano, salt, and pepper. Cook for a few more minutes until everything is well combined.
5. Arrange the bell peppers in a baking dish. Spoon the turkey and quinoa mixture into each bell pepper.
6. If using cheese, sprinkle it on top of the stuffed peppers.
7. Cover the baking dish with aluminum foil and bake for 25-30 minutes or until the peppers are tender.
8. Remove the foil and bake for an additional 5 minutes to melt the cheese if using.
9. Garnish with fresh parsley before serving.

Nutritional Facts:
- Calories: 320
- Total Fat: 12g
- Total Carbs: 25g
- Fiber: 5g
- Net Carbs: 20g
- Protein: 28g

Cooking Tip: *For a vegetarian version, replace the ground turkey with black beans or lentils. You can also add other vegetables like corn, spinach, or mushrooms to the filling. For a spicier flavor, include diced jalapeños or chili powder. These stuffed peppers can be prepared in advance and baked just before serving. They also reheat well for leftovers.*

Recipe 34: Eggplant Parmesan

Prep Time: 20 mins - Cooking Time: 30 mins - Serves: 4

Ingredients:
2 large eggplants, sliced into 1/2-inch rounds
Salt
2 cups breadcrumbs
1 teaspoon Italian seasoning
1/2 cup grated Parmesan cheese
2 eggs, beaten
3 cups marinara sauce
2 cups shredded mozzarella cheese
Olive oil for brushing
Fresh basil for garnish

Instructions:
1. Preheat the oven to 375°F (190°C). Place the eggplant slices in a colander, sprinkle with salt, and let them sit for about 15 minutes to draw out moisture.
2. In a shallow bowl, combine the breadcrumbs, Italian seasoning, and grated Parmesan cheese.
3. In another shallow bowl, beat the eggs.
4. Rinse the eggplant slices and pat them dry with paper towels.
5. Dip each eggplant slice first in the beaten egg, then in the breadcrumb mixture, coating both sides.
6. Place the breaded eggplant slices on a baking sheet lined with parchment paper. Brush each slice lightly with olive oil.
7. Bake for 15 minutes, then flip the slices and bake for another 15 minutes or until they are golden brown and crispy.
8. In a baking dish, spread a layer of marinara sauce. Place a layer of baked eggplant slices over the sauce. Top with more marinara sauce and a layer of shredded mozzarella cheese.
9. Repeat the layers until all ingredients are used, finishing with a cheese layer.
10. Bake in the oven for 20-30 minutes or until the cheese is melted and bubbly.
11. Garnish with fresh basil before serving.

Nutritional Facts:
- Calories: 450
- Total Fat: 20g
- Total Carbs: 45g
- Fiber: 9g
- Net Carbs: 36g
- Protein: 25g

Cooking Tip: *For a lighter version, you can grill or broil the eggplant slices instead of breading and baking them. You can also use whole wheat breadcrumbs for a healthier alternative. For a gluten-free version, use gluten-free breadcrumbs. This dish can be made ahead and reheated, making it a great option for meal prep or entertaining.*

Recipe 35: Pork Tenderloin with Apple Cider Glaze

Prep Time: 20 mins - Cooking Time: 30 mins - Serves: 4

Ingredients:
1 pork tenderloin (about 1 to 1.5 pounds)
Salt and pepper to taste
2 tablespoons olive oil
1 cup apple cider
2 tablespoons apple cider vinegar
2 tablespoons honey or brown sugar
1 teaspoon Dijon mustard
2 cloves garlic, minced
1/2 teaspoon dried thyme
Assorted root vegetables (such as carrots, parsnips, and potatoes), peeled and cut into chunks

Instructions:
1. Preheat the oven to 375°F (190°C).
2. Season the pork tenderloin with salt and pepper.
3. Heat 1 tablespoon of olive oil in a large ovenproof skillet over medium-high heat. Add the pork tenderloin and sear on all sides until golden brown, about 2-3 minutes per side.
4. In a bowl, whisk together the apple cider, apple cider vinegar, honey or brown sugar, Dijon mustard, minced garlic, and dried thyme to make the glaze.
5. Pour half of the glaze over the pork tenderloin in the skillet.
6. In a separate bowl, toss the root vegetables with the remaining 1 tablespoon of olive oil and a bit of salt and pepper. Arrange them around the pork in the skillet.
7. Roast in the oven for 25-30 minutes or until the pork reaches an internal temperature of 145°F (63°C). Baste the pork occasionally with the pan juices.
8. Remove the pork from the oven and let it rest for 5-10 minutes before slicing.
9. Serve the pork tenderloin slices with the roasted root vegetables and drizzle with the remaining apple cider glaze.

Nutritional Facts:
- Calories: 410
- Total Fat: 14g
- Total Carbs: 30g
- Fiber: 3g
- Net Carbs: 27g
- Protein: 40g

Cooking Tip: *For a deeper flavor, add a splash of bourbon to the glaze. You can also include herbs like rosemary or sage for added aroma. The root vegetables can be pre-roasted for 10-15 minutes before adding the pork if you prefer them to be more cooked. This dish pairs well with a side of green beans or a simple salad.*

Recipe 36: Vegetarian Black Bean Enchiladas

Prep Time: 20 mins - Cooking Time: 25 mins - Serves: 4

Ingredients:
For the Enchiladas:
8 flour tortillas
2 cans (15 ounces each) black beans, drained and rinsed
1 cup corn kernels, fresh or frozen
2 cups shredded cheese (such as cheddar or Mexican blend) divided
1/2 red onion, chopped
1 teaspoon ground cumin
1/2 teaspoon chili powder
Salt and pepper to taste

For the Enchilada Sauce:
2 tablespoons vegetable oil
2 tablespoons all-purpose flour
1 tablespoon chili powder
2 cups vegetable broth
1 can (8 ounces) tomato sauce
1 teaspoon cumin
1/2 teaspoon garlic powder
Salt to taste

Instructions:
1. Preheat the oven to 375°F (190°C).
2. To make the enchilada sauce, heat the oil in a saucepan over medium heat. Stir in the flour and chili powder and cook for 1 minute.
3. Gradually whisk in the vegetable broth, ensuring there are no lumps. Add the tomato sauce, cumin, and garlic powder. Bring to a simmer and cook until the sauce thickens about 5 minutes. Season with salt.
4. In a bowl, mix together the black beans, corn, half of the cheese, red onion, ground cumin, chili powder, salt, and pepper.
5. Spread a little enchilada sauce on the bottom of a baking dish.
6. Fill each tortilla with the bean mixture, roll it up, and place seam-side down in the baking dish.
7. Pour the remaining enchilada sauce over the rolled tortillas and sprinkle with the remaining cheese.
8. Bake in the preheated oven for 25 minutes or until the sauce is bubbly and the cheese is melted.
9. Serve the enchiladas hot, optionally garnished with fresh cilantro, diced avocado, or sour cream.

Nutritional Facts:
- Calories: 520
- Total Fat: 20g
- Total Carbs: 70g
- Fiber: 15g
- Net Carbs: 55g
- Protein: 20g

Cooking Tip: *For a gluten-free version, use corn tortillas instead of flour tortillas. You can also add other vegetables like bell peppers or spinach to the bean mixture. For a spicier enchilada, include diced jalapeños in the filling or use a hot enchilada sauce. These enchiladas can be assembled ahead of time and baked just before serving.*

Chapter 14: Guilt-Free Pleasures - Snacks & Desserts

This chapter is about snacks and desserts, showing that you can enjoy indulgence while still maintaining a diet. It offers a variety of snack ideas and dessert recipes that are both delicious for you and perfect for satisfying those cravings. These treats are designed to be guilt-free and align with the principles of fasting.

Recipe 37: Crispy Baked Apple Chips: Apples are baked to perfection until they turn crispy, with a touch of cinnamon added for a naturally sweet and healthy snack.

Recipe 38: Decadent Dark Chocolate Avocado Truffles: truffles made with avocado and rich dark chocolate rolled in cocoa powder to create a luxurious yet wholesome treat.

Recipe 39: Refreshing Greek Yogurt and Berry Frozen Bars: Bars made with Greek yogurt, mixed berries, and a drizzle of honey provide a refreshing snack option.

Recipe 40: Quick No Bake Peanut Butter Oat Balls: Energy-boosting balls prepared using oats, peanut butter, and flax seeds; perfect for when you need a satisfying snack.

Recipe 41: Zucchini and Parmesan Muffins: Flavorful muffins packed with zucchini and Parmesan cheese; an excellent choice for those seeking a savory snack.

Recipe 42: Crunchy Roasted Chickpeas, with Smoked Paprika: Crispy chickpeas roasted in olive oil infused with smoked paprika; a protein snack option.

Recipe 43: Raspberry Chia Seed Pudding: Indulge in a tangy pudding crafted from chia seeds, almond milk, and picked raspberries. This delightful treat is what you need for a refreshing dessert.

Recipe 44: Carrot Cake Energy Bites: Savor the goodness of these bites that capture the essence of carrot cake without any guilt. They are expertly crafted with carrots, a medley of nuts, and a blend of spices.

Recipe 45: Almond Butter and Banana Frozen Yogurt Bark: Experience the delight of yogurt bark adorned with delightful swirls of almond butter and luscious slices of banana. It's truly an effortless snack option when you're on the go.

Recipe 46: Baked Cinnamon Pear Slices: Treat yourself to the simplicity and natural sweetness of succulent pear slices baked to perfection with a hint of cinnamon and nutmeg. This makes for a snack.

Recipe 47: Pumpkin Spice Protein Smoothie: Embark on a journey with this smoothie that harmoniously blends pumpkin puree, ripe bananas, protein powder, and tantalizing pumpkin spice. It's a workout indulgence.

Recipe 48: Coconut and Almond Date Balls: Delight your taste buds with these balls made from dates infused with tropical coconut goodness and crunchy almonds. They provide the solution when those sweet cravings strike.

Recipe 37: Baked Apple Chips

Prep Time: 10 mins - Cooking Time: 2-3 hrs - Serves: 4

Ingredients:

2 large apples (such as Fuji, Gala, or Honeycrisp)

Ground cinnamon to taste

Optional: A sprinkle of sugar or sugar substitute

Instructions:

1. Preheat the oven to 200°F (95°C). Line two baking sheets with parchment paper.

2. Wash the apples and slice them very thinly, using a mandoline slicer for consistent thickness. Remove any seeds.

3. Arrange the apple slices in a single layer on the prepared baking sheets.

4. Sprinkle the apple slices lightly with cinnamon and sugar or sugar substitute if using.

5. Bake in the preheated oven for 1 hour. Flip the apple slices and continue baking for another 1-2 hours or until they are crisp and no longer moist.

6. Keep an eye on them to ensure they do not burn, especially if your oven runs hot.

7. Once done, turn off the oven and let the apple chips cool inside for 1 hour to crisp up further.

8. Store the apple chips in an airtight container.

Nutritional Facts:

- Calories (per serving): 50

- Total Fat: 0g

- Total Carbs: 13g

- Fiber: 2g

- Net Carbs: 11g

- Protein: 0g

Cooking Tip: Make sure the apple slices are as thin as possible for the best results. You can also experiment with different spices like nutmeg or pumpkin spice for a variety. Baking times may vary based on the thickness of the slices and the moisture content of the apples, so it's important to keep an eye on them, particularly towards the end of the baking time. These apple chips are a great healthy snack on their own or can be used as a topping for yogurt or oatmeal.

Recipe 38: Dark Chocolate Avocado Truffles

Prep Time: 20 mins - Chill Time: 1 hr - Makes: 12-15 truffles

Ingredients:
2 ripe avocados, pitted and peeled
8 ounces dark chocolate, chopped (70% cocoa or higher)
1 tablespoon honey or maple syrup (optional for sweetness)
1 teaspoon vanilla extract
A pinch of salt
1/4 cup cocoa powder for rolling
Optional: Finely chopped nuts or shredded coconut for coating

Instructions:
1. Melt the dark chocolate in a heatproof bowl over a pot of simmering water (double boiler) or in the microwave in 30-second intervals, stirring until smooth.
2. In a food processor, blend the ripe avocados until smooth.
3. Add the melted chocolate, honey, or maple syrup (if using), vanilla extract, and a pinch of salt to the blended avocado. Process until the mixture is well combined and creamy.
4. Transfer the chocolate avocado mixture to a bowl and refrigerate for about 30 minutes or until it's firm enough to handle.
5. Using a spoon or melon baller, scoop out small portions of the mixture and roll into balls with your hands.
6. Place the cocoa powder in a shallow dish (and any other coatings like chopped nuts or shredded coconut, if using). Roll the truffles in the cocoa powder until fully coated.
7. Place the truffles on a plate or baking sheet lined with parchment paper.
8. Refrigerate the truffles for at least 30 minutes before serving to set.

Nutritional Facts (per truffle):
- Calories: 120
- Total Fat: 9g
- Total Carbs: 10g
- Fiber: 3g
- Net Carbs: 7g
- Protein: 2g

***Cooking Tip:** Ensure the avocados are well-ripened for the best texture. For a vegan version, choose vegan dark chocolate and maple syrup as a sweetener. These truffles can be stored in an airtight container in the refrigerator for up to a week. For a different flavor profile, you can add a splash of rum, orange zest, or a pinch of chili powder to the truffle mixture.*

Recipe 39: Greek Yogurt and Berry Frozen Bars

Prep Time: 15 mins - Freeze Time: 4 hrs - Makes: 8-10 bars

Ingredients:
2 cups Greek yogurt
1/4 cup honey or maple syrup, plus more for drizzling
1 teaspoon vanilla extract
1 1/2 cups mixed berries (such as strawberries, blueberries, raspberries)
Optional: Chopped nuts or granola for texture

Instructions:
1. In a bowl, mix together the Greek yogurt, 1/4 cup of honey or maple syrup, and vanilla extract until well combined.
2. If using, fold the chopped nuts or granola into the yogurt mixture for added crunch.
3. Gently fold in the mixed berries, being careful not to crush them.
4. Line a baking dish or a loaf pan with parchment paper, leaving some overhang on the sides for easy removal.
5. Pour the yogurt and berry mixture into the prepared dish and smooth the top with a spatula.
6. Drizzle additional honey or maple syrup over the top.
7. Place the dish in the freezer and freeze for at least 4 hours or until the mixture is firm.
8. Once frozen, lift the frozen yogurt mixture out of the dish using the parchment paper overhang and place it on a cutting board.
9. Cut into bars or squares using a sharp knife.
10. Serve the Greek yogurt and berry frozen bars immediately as a refreshing and healthy snack.

Nutritional Facts (per bar):
- Calories: 120
- Total Fat: 2g
- Total Carbs: 18g
- Fiber: 2g
- Net Carbs: 16g
- Protein: 8g

***Cooking Tip**: For a smoother texture, you can blend the berries with some of the yogurt before folding it into the rest of the mixture. You can also layer the yogurt and berries for a striped effect. These bars can be customized with your favorite fruits and additional toppings like chocolate chips or coconut flakes. Store the bars in the freezer in an airtight container with parchment paper between them to prevent sticking.*

Recipe 40: No-Bake Peanut Butter Oat Balls

Prep Time: 15 mins - Chill Time: 30 mins - Makes: 12-15 balls

Ingredients:

1 cup rolled oats
1/2 cup natural peanut butter
1/4 cup honey or maple syrup
1/4 cup ground flax seeds
1/2 teaspoon vanilla extract
Optional: Mini chocolate chips, chopped nuts, or dried fruit

Instructions:

1. In a large bowl, combine the rolled oats, peanut butter, honey or maple syrup, and ground flax seeds. Mix until well combined.

2. Add the vanilla extract and stir again. If using, fold in the mini chocolate chips, chopped nuts, or dried fruit for added flavor and texture.

3. Using your hands, roll the mixture into small balls about 1 inch in diameter.

4. Place the oat balls on a baking sheet lined with parchment paper or in a container.

5. Refrigerate the oat balls for at least 30 minutes to set.

6. Once set, transfer the peanut butter oat balls to an airtight container and store them in the refrigerator.

Nutritional Facts (per ball):

- Calories: 110
- Total Fat: 6g
- Total Carbs: 12g
- Fiber: 2g
- Net Carbs: 10g
- Protein: 3g

Cooking Tip: *For a vegan version, use maple syrup instead of honey. To add more protein to these balls, include a scoop of your favorite protein powder. If the mixture is too dry, add a bit more peanut butter or honey. For a different flavor, you can substitute almond butter or cashew butter for the peanut butter. These no-bake oat balls are great for meal prep and can be stored in the refrigerator for up to a week or in the freezer for longer.*

Recipe 41: Zucchini and Parmesan Savory Muffins

Prep Time: 15 mins - Cooking Time: 20 mins - Makes: 12 muffins

Ingredients:
2 cups all-purpose flour
1 tablespoon baking powder
1/2 teaspoon baking soda
1/2 teaspoon salt
1/4 teaspoon black pepper
1 cup grated zucchini (excess moisture squeezed out)
1 cup grated Parmesan cheese
1/4 cup olive oil
1 cup buttermilk or milk
2 large eggs
2 tablespoons chopped fresh herbs (such as parsley, chives, or basil)

Instructions:
1. Preheat the oven to 375°F (190°C). Grease or line a 12-cup muffin tin with paper liners.
2. In a large bowl, whisk together the flour, baking powder, baking soda, salt, and black pepper.
3. Stir in the grated zucchini and Parmesan cheese.
4. In another bowl, whisk together the olive oil, buttermilk or milk, and eggs.
5. Add the wet ingredients to the dry ingredients and mix until just combined. Be careful not to overmix.
6. Gently fold in the chopped fresh herbs.
7. Spoon the batter into the prepared muffin tin, filling each cup about 3/4 full.
8. Bake in the preheated oven for 20 minutes or until the muffins are golden brown and a toothpick inserted into the center comes out clean.
9. Remove the muffins from the oven and let them cool in the tin for a few minutes before transferring them to a wire rack to cool completely.

Nutritional Facts (per muffin):
- Calories: 180
- Total Fat: 9g
- Total Carbs: 18g
- Fiber: 1g
- Net Carbs: 17g
- Protein: 7g

Cooking Tip: For a healthier version, you can use whole wheat flour instead of all-purpose flour. You can also add other vegetables, like finely chopped bell peppers or sun-dried tomatoes, for extra flavor. If you don't have buttermilk, you can make your own by adding a tablespoon of lemon juice or vinegar to a cup of milk and letting it sit for 5 minutes. These muffins can be stored in an airtight container for up to 3 days or frozen for longer storage.

Recipe 42: Roasted Chickpeas with Smoked Paprika

Prep Time: 5 mins - Cooking Time: 30-40 mins - Serves: 4

Ingredients:

2 cans (15 ounces each) chickpeas, drained, rinsed, and patted dry
2 tablespoons olive oil
1 1/2 teaspoons smoked paprika
Salt to taste
Optional: Ground cumin, garlic powder, or chili powder for additional flavor

Instructions:

1. Preheat the oven to 400°F (200°C). Line a baking sheet with parchment paper.

2. In a bowl, toss the dried chickpeas with olive oil, smoked paprika, and salt until evenly coated. If using additional spices like cumin, garlic powder, or chili powder, add them to the mix.

3. Spread the chickpeas in a single layer on the prepared baking sheet.

4. Roast in the preheated oven for 30-40 minutes or until the chickpeas are crispy and golden brown. Stir them a few times during cooking to ensure even roasting.

5. Remove from the oven and let the chickpeas cool slightly; they will continue to crisp up as they cool.

6. Serve the roasted chickpeas warm or at room temperature as a crunchy, protein-rich snack.

Nutritional Facts (per serving):

- Calories: 210
- Total Fat: 8g
- Total Carbs: 27g
- Fiber: 8g
- Net Carbs: 19g
- Protein: 10g

Cooking Tip: *To achieve the crispiest chickpeas, ensure they are thoroughly dried after rinsing. You can experiment with different seasonings and spices according to your preference. Roasted chickpeas are best enjoyed the same day, as they lose their crispiness over time. If you have leftovers, you can re-crisp them in the oven for a few minutes before serving. These make a great addition to salads or as a topping for soups.*

Recipe 43: Raspberry Chia Seed Pudding

Prep Time: 10 mins - Chill Time: 4 hrs or overnight - Serves: 4

Ingredients:

1/4 cup chia seeds
1 cup almond milk (or any milk of your choice)
1 cup fresh raspberries
2 tablespoons honey or maple syrup
1/2 teaspoon vanilla extract
Additional raspberries and mint leaves for garnish (optional)

Instructions:

1. In a mixing bowl, combine the chia seeds and almond milk. Stir well.

2. Mash the raspberries with a fork and add them to the chia mixture. You can leave some whole raspberries for texture or puree them for a smoother pudding.

3. Add honey or maple syrup and vanilla extract to the mixture. Mix until all the ingredients are well combined.

4. Divide the mixture into four serving glasses or jars. Cover and refrigerate for at least 4 hours or overnight until the pudding has thickened and the chia seeds have absorbed the liquid.

5. Before serving, stir the pudding to ensure an even texture. If the pudding is too thick, you can add a little more almond milk to reach your desired consistency.

6. Garnish with additional fresh raspberries and mint leaves, if desired.

7. Serve the chilled raspberry chia seed pudding as a refreshing and healthy dessert or snack.

Nutritional Facts (per serving):

- Calories: 140
- Total Fat: 5g
- Total Carbs: 21g
- Fiber: 7g
- Net Carbs: 14g
- Protein: 4g

***Cooking Tip:** For a creamier pudding, you can blend the raspberries and almond milk together before mixing with the chia seeds. You can also layer the pudding with granola, nuts, or coconut flakes for added texture. This pudding can be stored in the refrigerator for up to 5 days, making it a great option for meal prep. For a vegan version, ensure to use maple syrup or a vegan sweetener.*

Recipe 44: Carrot Cake Energy Bites

Prep Time: 20 mins - No Cooking - Makes: 12-15 bites

Ingredients:

1 cup rolled oats
1/2 cup grated carrots
1/2 cup dates, pitted and chopped
1/2 cup walnuts or pecans, chopped
1/4 cup shredded coconut
2 tablespoons honey or maple syrup
1 teaspoon ground cinnamon
1/2 teaspoon ground ginger
1/4 teaspoon ground nutmeg
1/4 teaspoon salt
Optional: 1/4 cup raisins or dried cranberries

Instructions:

1. In a food processor, combine the rolled oats, grated carrots, chopped dates, walnuts or pecans, and shredded coconut. Pulse until the mixture is well combined, and the dates are finely chopped.

2. Add the honey or maple syrup, cinnamon, ginger, nutmeg, and salt. Pulse again until the mixture starts to come together and form a sticky dough.

3. If using, fold in the raisins or dried cranberries by hand.

4. Using your hands, roll the mixture into small balls about 1 inch in diameter.

5. Place the carrot cake energy bites on a plate or tray lined with parchment paper.

6. Refrigerate the bites for at least 30 minutes to firm up.

7. Store the energy bites in an airtight container in the refrigerator.

Nutritional Facts (per bite):

- Calories: 100
- Total Fat: 5g
- Total Carbs: 13g
- Fiber: 2g
- Net Carbs: 11g
- Protein: 2g

Cooking Tip: *For a nut-free version, you can substitute the nuts with sunflower seeds or pumpkin seeds. If the mixture is too dry, add a little more honey or maple syrup. You can also coat the energy bites in additional shredded coconut or finely chopped nuts for extra texture. These bites are perfect for a quick snack, a post-workout boost, or a healthy treat on the go.*

Recipe 45: Almond Butter and Banana Frozen Yogurt Bark

Prep Time: 10 mins - Freeze Time: 2-3 hrs - Makes: Several pieces

Ingredients:
2 cups Greek yogurt
1/4 cup honey or maple syrup
1/2 teaspoon vanilla extract
1/4 cup almond butter, slightly warmed for drizzling
2 ripe bananas, sliced
Optional: Chopped nuts, chocolate chips, or shredded coconut for topping

Instructions:
1. In a bowl, mix the Greek yogurt with honey or maple syrup and vanilla extract until well combined.
2. Line a baking sheet with parchment paper.
3. Spread the yogurt mixture evenly onto the lined baking sheet, about 1/4 inch thick.
4. Drizzle the almond butter over the yogurt. Use a toothpick or knife to gently swirl the almond butter into the yogurt.
5. Arrange the banana slices over the yogurt layer. Press them down slightly into the yogurt.
6. If using, sprinkle the top with chopped nuts, chocolate chips, or shredded coconut.
7. Place the baking sheet in the freezer and freeze for 2-3 hours or until the yogurt is fully set and firm.
8. Once frozen, break the yogurt bark into pieces of your desired size.
9. Serve immediately or store the frozen yogurt bark in an airtight container in the freezer.

Nutritional Facts (per serving, varies by size):
- Calories: 120 (approx.)
- Total Fat: 5g (approx.)
- Total Carbs: 15g (approx.)
- Fiber: 1g (approx.)
- Net Carbs: 14g (approx.)
- Protein: 6g (approx.)

Cooking Tip: For a vegan version, use plant-based yogurt and maple syrup. The almond butter can be substituted with peanut butter or any other nut butter of your choice. For added texture and flavor, you can also incorporate a layer of granola before freezing. This treat is perfect for hot days and can be a great way to get kids to enjoy a healthy snack.

Recipe 46: Baked Cinnamon Pear Slices

Prep Time: 10 mins - Cooking Time: 25 mins - Serves: 4

Ingredients:

4 ripe pears, cored and sliced
2 tablespoons honey or maple syrup
1 teaspoon ground cinnamon
1/4 teaspoon ground nutmeg
A pinch of salt
Optional: A sprinkle of granulated sugar for extra sweetness

Instructions:

1. Preheat the oven to 350°F (175°C). Line a baking sheet with parchment paper.

2. Arrange the pear slices in a single layer on the prepared baking sheet.

3. In a small bowl, mix together the honey or maple syrup, cinnamon, nutmeg, and a pinch of salt.

4. Brush the mixture over the pear slices, coating them evenly. If using, sprinkle a little granulated sugar on top for added sweetness.

5. Bake in the preheated oven for 25 minutes or until the pear slices are tender and lightly caramelized.

6. Remove from the oven and let cool slightly.

7. Serve the baked cinnamon pear slices as a warm snack dessert or as a topping for yogurt or oatmeal.

Nutritional Facts (per serving):

- Calories: 120
- Total Fat: 0g
- Total Carbs: 30g
- Fiber: 5g
- Net Carbs: 25g
- Protein: 1g

Cooking Tip: *Choose pears that are ripe but still firm for the best texture. You can also add a splash of lemon juice to the honey mixture to prevent the pears from browning and to add a tangy flavor. For a different variation, try using different spices like cardamom or ginger. These baked pear slices can also be served with a scoop of vanilla ice cream or a dollop of whipped cream for an indulgent treat.*

Recipe 47: Pumpkin Spice Protein Smoothie

Prep Time: 5 mins - No Cooking - Serves: 2

Ingredients:

1 cup pumpkin puree (canned or fresh)
1 ripe banana
1 scoop vanilla protein powder
1 1/2 cups almond milk or milk of choice
1 tablespoon honey or maple syrup (optional, depending on sweetness preference)
1 teaspoon pumpkin pie spice (or a mix of cinnamon, nutmeg, ginger, and allspice)
1/2 teaspoon vanilla extract
Ice cubes (optional for a thicker smoothie)

Instructions:

1. In a blender, combine the pumpkin puree, ripe banana, vanilla protein powder, almond milk, honey, or maple syrup (if using), pumpkin pie spice, and vanilla extract.

2. Add a handful of ice cubes if you prefer a thicker consistency.

3. Blend on high speed until the mixture is smooth and creamy.

4. Taste and adjust the sweetness or spices as needed.

5. Pour the smoothie into glasses and serve immediately.

Nutritional Facts (per serving):

- Calories: 220
- Total Fat: 3g
- Total Carbs: 35g
- Fiber: 5g
- Net Carbs: 30g
- Protein: 15g

Cooking Tip: *For an extra nutritional boost, you can add a tablespoon of flax seeds or chia seeds. If you don't have pumpkin pie spice, you can make your own by mixing equal parts of ground cinnamon, nutmeg, ginger, and allspice. To make the smoothie more filling, you can add a tablespoon of almond butter or oats. This pumpkin spice protein smoothie is perfect for autumn mornings or as a nutritious snack any time of the year.*

Recipe 48: Coconut and Almond Date Balls

Prep Time: 15 mins - No Cooking - Makes: 12-15 balls

Ingredients:

1 cup Medjool dates, pitted
1/2 cup raw almonds
1/2 cup shredded unsweetened coconut, plus extra for coating
1 teaspoon vanilla extract
A pinch of salt
Optional: 1 tablespoon of cocoa powder or a few drops of almond extract for extra flavor

Instructions:

1. In a food processor, add the pitted dates and raw almonds. Process until they form a sticky, crumbly mixture.

2. Add the shredded coconut, vanilla extract, and a pinch of salt to the date and almond mixture. If using, add cocoa powder or almond extract. Process again until all ingredients are well combined, and the mixture sticks together when pressed.

3. Take small portions of the mixture and roll them into balls about 1 inch in diameter.

4. Roll each ball in additional shredded coconut until coated on all sides.

5. Place the coconut and almond date balls on a plate or tray.

6. Refrigerate for at least 30 minutes to firm up before serving.

7. Store the date balls in an airtight container in the refrigerator.

Nutritional Facts (per ball):

- Calories: 100
- Total Fat: 5g
- Total Carbs: 15g
- Fiber: 3g
- Net Carbs: 12g
- Protein: 2g

Cooking Tip: *Soaking the dates in warm water for 10 minutes before processing can make them easier to blend, especially if they are a bit dry. You can substitute almonds with other nuts like cashews or walnuts. These balls can also be rolled in chopped nuts, cocoa powder, or sesame seeds for variety. They are a great energy booster and a healthier alternative to traditional sweets.*

Chapter 15: Complementary Flavors - Side Recipes

In this chapter, we will explore a range of side dishes that perfectly complement any course. These recipes offer a mix of vegetables and creative grain-based dishes, ensuring both variety and nutritional value in your meals. They are crafted to be simple yet packed with flavor, enhancing the dining experience while focusing on suitable ingredients for fasting.

Recipe 49: Roasted Brussels Sprouts with Garlic: Enjoy the crispy and golden goodness of Brussels sprouts roasted with olive oil. This dish serves as an accompaniment to any meal.

Recipe 50: Quinoa Tabbouleh Twist: Experience a twist on tabbouleh by replacing bulgur with quinoa. Combined with tomatoes, cucumber, and a zesty herb dressing, it offers a burst of flavor.

Recipe 51: Sweet and Tangy Balsamic Glazed Baby Carrots: Treat your taste buds to tender baby carrots coated in a tangy balsamic reduction. This dish adds an explosion of flavor to any plate.

Recipe 52: Lemon Herb Couscous: Indulge in fluffy couscous infused with the freshness of lemon juice and fragrant herbs. This versatile side pairs beautifully with dishes.

Recipe 53: Almond-topped Steamed Green Beans: Delight in steamed beans adorned with toasted almonds and a subtle hint of lemon zest.

Recipe 54: Roasted Beet Salad with Creamy Goat Cheese: Discover the blend of roasted beets, creamy goat cheese, and a drizzle of tangy balsamic vinaigrette. This salad brightens up any meal.

Recipe 55:. Cilantro Lime Rice: Fragrant rice side dish infused with the flavors of fresh cilantro and zesty lime juice, perfect for enhancing Mexican or Asian cuisines.

Recipe 56: Spiced Sweet Potato Wedges: Baked sweet potato wedges seasoned with a blend of spices, offering a twist on traditional fries.

Recipe 57: Creamy Polenta: Smooth and velvety polenta, versatile side that can be customized with cheeses or herbs.

Recipe 58: Sautéed Spinach with Garlic: Quickly sautéed spinach leaves with a touch of garlic and olive oil, a way to savor your greens.

Recipe 59: Cauliflower Rice Pilaf: A carb alternative to rice pilaf using cauliflower "rice" combined with onions, garlic, and aromatic herbs.

Recipe 60: Grilled Asparagus with Lemon Butter: Grilled asparagus spears drizzled with a lemon butter sauce are an effortless addition to any meal.

Recipe 49: Garlic Roasted Brussels Sprouts

Prep Time: 10 mins - Cooking Time: 25 mins - Serves: 4

Ingredients:

1 pound Brussels sprouts, trimmed and halved

3 tablespoons olive oil

3-4 garlic cloves, minced

Salt and pepper to taste

Optional: Lemon juice or balsamic vinegar for finishing

Instructions:

1. Preheat the oven to 400°F (200°C). Line a baking sheet with parchment paper.

2. In a large bowl, toss the Brussels sprouts with olive oil, minced garlic, salt, and pepper until evenly coated.

3. Spread the Brussels sprouts in a single layer on the prepared baking sheet, ensuring they are not overcrowded.

4. Roast in the preheated oven for 20-25 minutes or until the Brussels sprouts are crispy on the outside and tender on the inside. Stir them halfway through the cooking time for even roasting.

5. Remove from the oven. Optionally, sprinkle a little lemon juice or drizzle balsamic vinegar over the Brussels sprouts for added flavor.

6. Serve the garlic-roasted Brussels sprouts immediately as a delicious and healthy side dish.

Nutritional Facts (per serving):

- Calories: 130
- Total Fat: 10g
- Total Carbs: 10g
- Fiber: 4g
- Net Carbs: 6g
- Protein: 3g

Cooking Tip: For extra crispiness, you can broil the Brussels sprouts for the last 2-3 minutes of cooking. Adding Parmesan cheese or crushed red pepper flakes can provide additional flavor. You can also mix in other vegetables like carrots or sweet potatoes for a more colorful and varied side dish. This recipe is versatile and pairs well with a wide range of main courses, from grilled meats to vegetarian options.

Recipe 50: Quinoa Tabbouleh

Prep Time: 15 mins - Cooking Time: 15 mins - Serves: 4

Ingredients:

1 cup quinoa, rinsed and drained
2 cups water
1 cup cherry tomatoes, halved
1 cucumber, diced
1/4 cup red onion, finely chopped
1/2 cup fresh parsley, finely chopped
1/4 cup fresh mint, finely chopped
Juice of 2 lemons
1/4 cup olive oil
Salt and pepper to taste

Instructions:

1. In a saucepan, bring the quinoa and water to a boil. Reduce the heat to low, cover, and simmer for about 15 minutes, or until the quinoa is cooked and the water is absorbed.

2. Fluff the cooked quinoa with a fork and let it cool to room temperature.

3. In a large bowl, combine the cooled quinoa, cherry tomatoes, cucumber, red onion, parsley, and mint.

4. In a small bowl, whisk together the lemon juice, olive oil, salt, and pepper to create the dressing.

5. Pour the dressing over the quinoa salad and toss gently to combine all the ingredients.

6. Adjust the seasoning with additional salt and pepper if needed.

7. Refrigerate the tabbouleh for at least 30 minutes before serving to allow the flavors to meld.

8. Serve the quinoa tabbouleh chilled as a refreshing side dish or light meal.

Nutritional Facts (per serving):

- Calories: 280
- Total Fat: 14g
- Total Carbs: 33g
- Fiber: 5g
- Net Carbs: 28g
- Protein: 7g

Cooking Tip: *For added crunch and flavor, you can include diced bell pepper or radishes. You can also add a sprinkle of feta cheese or olives for a Mediterranean twist. This dish can be stored in the refrigerator for up to 3 days, making it a great option for meal prep. For a gluten-free version, make sure to use certified gluten-free quinoa.*

Recipe 51: Balsamic Glazed Baby Carrots

Prep Time: 5 mins - Cooking Time: 25 mins - Serves: 4

Ingredients:

1 pound baby carrots, washed and dried

2 tablespoons olive oil

Salt and pepper to taste

1/4 cup balsamic vinegar

2 tablespoons honey or brown sugar

Optional: Fresh thyme or parsley for garnish

Instructions:

1. Preheat the oven to 400°F (200°C).

2. In a bowl, toss the baby carrots with olive oil, salt, and pepper.

3. Spread the carrots in a single layer on a baking sheet and roast in the oven for 20 minutes or until they are tender and starting to caramelize.

4. While the carrots are roasting, prepare the balsamic glaze. In a small saucepan, combine the balsamic vinegar and honey or brown sugar. Bring to a simmer over medium heat and cook until the mixture reduces by half and thickens into a syrupy glaze, about 5 minutes.

5. Once the carrots are roasted, remove them from the oven and drizzle the balsamic glaze over them. Toss gently to coat all the carrots evenly.

6. Return the carrots to the oven for an additional 5 minutes to glaze.

7. Serve the balsamic glazed baby carrots warm, garnished with fresh thyme or parsley if desired.

Nutritional Facts (per serving):

- Calories: 140
- Total Fat: 7g
- Total Carbs: 19g
- Fiber: 3g
- Net Carbs: 16g
- Protein: 1g

***Cooking Tip:** For added flavor, you can roast the carrots with a sprinkle of garlic powder or add a splash of orange juice to the balsamic glaze. You can also experiment with different types of vinegar, like red wine vinegar or apple cider vinegar, for a different twist. This dish is a great accompaniment to a variety of main courses, from roasted meats to vegetarian entrees.*

Recipe 52: Lemon Herb Couscous

Prep Time: 5 mins - Cooking Time: 10 mins - Serves: 4

Ingredients:

1 cup couscous

1 1/4 cups water or vegetable broth

1 tablespoon olive oil

Juice and zest of 1 lemon

1/4 cup fresh parsley, finely chopped

1/4 cup fresh mint, finely chopped

Salt and pepper to taste

Optional: 2 tablespoons toasted pine nuts or slivered almonds

Instructions:

1. In a saucepan, bring the water or vegetable broth to a boil. Add the olive oil and a pinch of salt.

2. Stir in the couscous and remove the saucepan from heat. Cover and let it sit for 5 minutes, allowing the couscous to absorb the liquid and become fluffy.

3. Fluff the couscous with a fork to break up any clumps.

4. Add the lemon juice, lemon zest, chopped parsley, and mint to the couscous. Gently mix to combine all the ingredients.

5. Season with salt and pepper to taste.

6. If using, sprinkle toasted pine nuts or slivered almonds over the couscous for added crunch and flavor.

7. Serve the lemon herb couscous warm or at room temperature as a light and versatile side dish.

Nutritional Facts (per serving):

- Calories: 200
- Total Fat: 4g
- Total Carbs: 35g
- Fiber: 2g
- Net Carbs: 33g
- Protein: 6g

Cooking Tip: *You can add additional herbs like cilantro or dill for different flavor profiles. For a heartier dish, mix in some chopped vegetables like bell peppers, tomatoes, or cucumbers. Lemon herb couscous can be served alongside grilled meats or fish or as part of a vegetarian meal. It's also great for meal prep as it keeps well in the refrigerator for a few days.*

Recipe 53: Steamed Green Beans with Almonds

Prep Time: 10 mins - Cooking Time: 10 mins - Serves: 4

Ingredients:

1 pound fresh green beans, trimmed
1/4 cup sliced almonds
2 tablespoons olive oil
Zest of 1 lemon
Salt and pepper to taste
Optional: A squeeze of fresh lemon juice, garlic powder, or crushed red pepper flakes for extra flavor

Instructions:

1. Steam the green beans until they are tender but still crisp, about 5 to 7 minutes. You can use a steaming basket over a pot of boiling water or a microwave steamer.

2. While the green beans are steaming, toast the sliced almonds in a dry skillet over medium heat. Stir frequently and watch closely to prevent burning until the almonds are golden brown and fragrant. Remove from heat.

3. Once the green beans are steamed, transfer them to a serving bowl.

4. Drizzle olive oil over the green beans and toss gently to coat.

5. Add the toasted almonds and lemon zest to the green beans. Toss again to distribute the almonds and zest evenly.

6. Season with salt and pepper to taste. If desired, add a squeeze of fresh lemon juice, a sprinkle of garlic powder, or a pinch of crushed red pepper flakes for extra flavor.

7. Serve the steamed green beans warm as a healthy and flavorful side dish.

Nutritional Facts (per serving):

- Calories: 130
- Total Fat: 9g
- Total Carbs: 10g
- Fiber: 4g
- Net Carbs: 6g
- Protein: 4g

Cooking Tip: For a richer flavor, you can sauté the steamed green beans with garlic in olive oil before adding the almonds and lemon zest. This dish pairs well with a variety of main courses, from grilled meats to baked fish. The green beans can also be blanched in boiling water for a few minutes and then shocked in ice water to retain their bright green color and crispness.

Recipe 54: Roasted Beet and Goat Cheese Salad

Prep Time: 15 mins - Cooking Time: 45 mins - Serves: 4

Ingredients:
4 medium beets, peeled and diced
2 tablespoons olive oil
Salt and pepper to taste
1/4 cup balsamic vinegar
1 teaspoon Dijon mustard
1 teaspoon honey or maple syrup
1/2 cup goat cheese, crumbled
Mixed salad greens (such as arugula or spinach)
Optional: Chopped walnuts or pecans, red onion slices

Instructions:
1. Preheat the oven to 400°F (200°C).
2. Toss the diced beets with 1 tablespoon of olive oil, salt, and pepper. Spread them on a baking sheet.
3. Roast the beets in the oven for about 45 minutes or until tender and slightly caramelized. Stir them occasionally for even cooking.
4. While the beets are roasting, prepare the dressing. Whisk together the balsamic vinegar, Dijon mustard, honey, or maple syrup, and the remaining 1 tablespoon of olive oil. Season with salt and pepper.
5. In a large salad bowl, combine the mixed greens with the roasted beets and crumbled goat cheese.
6. Drizzle the balsamic vinaigrette over the salad and toss gently to combine.
7. If using, top the salad with chopped nuts and red onion slices for added texture and flavor.
8. Serve the roasted beet and goat cheese salad immediately as a colorful and flavorful side dish or light meal.

Nutritional Facts (per serving):
- Calories: 220
- Total Fat: 14g
- Total Carbs: 16g
- Fiber: 4g
- Net Carbs: 12g
- Protein: 6g

Cooking Tip: *For added sweetness and contrast, you can add slices of orange or apple to the salad. Roasting the beets with a sprig of rosemary or thyme can infuse them with additional flavor. This salad can also be served with a sprinkle of fresh herbs like parsley or basil. The beets can be roasted in advance and stored in the refrigerator to save time.*

Recipe 55: Cilantro Lime Rice

Prep Time: 5 mins - Cooking Time: 20 mins - Serves: 4

Ingredients:

1 cup long-grain white rice
2 cups water
1/2 teaspoon salt
2 tablespoons olive oil
Juice and zest of 2 limes
1/4 cup fresh cilantro, finely chopped
Optional: 1 garlic clove, minced

Instructions:

1. Rinse the rice under cold water until the water runs clear. This helps to remove excess starch and prevents the rice from becoming too sticky.

2. In a saucepan, bring the water to a boil. Add the rinsed rice, salt, and olive oil. Stir once.

3. Reduce the heat to low, cover, and simmer for 18-20 minutes or until the water is absorbed and the rice is tender.

4. Remove the saucepan from the heat and let it sit, covered, for 5 minutes. This allows the rice to steam and become fluffy.

5. Fluff the rice with a fork to separate the grains. Stir in the lime juice, lime zest, and chopped cilantro. If using, add the minced garlic at this stage.

6. Adjust the seasoning, adding more salt or lime juice if needed.

7. Serve the cilantro lime rice warm as a vibrant and flavorful side dish perfect for pairing with Mexican or Asian dishes.

Nutritional Facts (per serving):

- Calories: 220
- Total Fat: 7g
- Total Carbs: 35g
- Fiber: 1g
- Net Carbs: 34g
- Protein: 3g

Cooking Tip: *For a different variation, you can cook the rice in chicken or vegetable broth instead of water for added flavor. Adding a bay leaf or a few whole peppercorns to the cooking water can also enhance the taste. If you prefer a little heat, a diced jalapeño can be added with the cilantro. This rice pairs well with dishes like tacos, burritos, grilled meats, or stir-fries. For a healthier version, you can use brown rice, but adjust the cooking time according to the package instructions.*

Recipe 56: Spiced Sweet Potato Wedges

Prep Time: 10 mins - Cooking Time: 30 mins - Serves: 4

Ingredients:

3 large sweet potatoes, cut into wedges
2 tablespoons olive oil
1 teaspoon smoked paprika
1/2 teaspoon garlic powder
1/2 teaspoon onion powder
1/4 teaspoon cayenne pepper (optional for heat)
Salt and pepper to taste
Optional: Fresh parsley or cilantro for garnish

Instructions:

1. Preheat the oven to 425°F (220°C). Line a baking sheet with parchment paper.

2. In a large bowl, toss the sweet potato wedges with olive oil, smoked paprika, garlic powder, onion powder, cayenne pepper (if using), salt, and pepper until evenly coated.

3. Spread the seasoned sweet potato wedges in a single layer on the prepared baking sheet, making sure they are not overcrowded.

4. Bake in the preheated oven for 30 minutes or until the wedges are tender and crispy on the edges. Flip the wedges halfway through the baking time for even cooking.

5. Remove from the oven and, if desired, garnish with fresh parsley or cilantro.

6. Serve the spiced sweet potato wedges warm as a tasty and healthier alternative to traditional fries.

Nutritional Facts (per serving):

- Calories: 220
- Total Fat: 7g
- Total Carbs: 37g
- Fiber: 6g
- Net Carbs: 31g
- Protein: 3g

Cooking Tip: *For extra crispiness, you can soak the cut sweet potatoes in cold water for 30 minutes before drying and seasoning them. This helps to remove excess starch. Feel free to experiment with other spices like ground cumin, curry powder, or dried herbs for different flavors. These wedges can be served with a dipping sauce like ketchup, aioli, or a yogurt-based dip. They make a great side dish for burgers, grilled meats, or as a part of a healthy snack spread.*

Recipe 57: Creamy Polenta

Prep Time: 5 mins - Cooking Time: 30 mins - Serves: 4

Ingredients:

1 cup polenta (coarse cornmeal)
4 cups water or chicken/vegetable broth
1 teaspoon salt
2 tablespoons butter
1/2 cup grated Parmesan cheese
Optional: Additional herbs like thyme or rosemary, more cheese like Gorgonzola or cheddar

Instructions:

1. In a large pot, bring the water or broth to a boil. Add the salt.

2. Gradually whisk in the polenta, ensuring to stir continuously to prevent lumps from forming.

3. Reduce the heat to low and continue to cook, stirring frequently, for about 25-30 minutes, or until the mixture thickens and the polenta is tender.

4. Once the polenta is cooked, stir in the butter and grated Parmesan cheese until well combined and creamy. If using, add your choice of additional herbs or cheese at this stage.

5. Taste and adjust the seasoning, adding more salt or cheese as needed.

6. Serve the creamy polenta hot as a side dish. It pairs well with braised meats, stews, or as a base for a variety of toppings.

Nutritional Facts (per serving):

- Calories: 260
- Total Fat: 10g
- Total Carbs: 34g
- Fiber: 2g
- Net Carbs: 32g
- Protein: 8g

Cooking Tip: *For a richer flavor, you can substitute half of the water or broth with milk or cream. To add more depth, consider sautéing some garlic or onion before adding the polenta. Creamy polenta can be served as it is or allowed to cool and then sliced and grilled or fried. This dish is a comforting base that can be adapted to suit a range of tastes and preferences.*

Recipe 58: Sautéed Spinach with Garlic

Prep Time: 5 mins - Cooking Time: 5 mins - Serves: 4

Ingredients:

2 tablespoons olive oil
4 garlic cloves, thinly sliced
1 pound fresh spinach leaves, washed and dried
Salt and pepper to taste
Optional: A squeeze of lemon juice or a sprinkle of red pepper flakes for extra flavor

Instructions:

1. Heat the olive oil in a large skillet over medium heat.

2. Add the sliced garlic and sauté for about 1 minute or until fragrant but not browned.

3. Increase the heat to medium-high and add the spinach leaves to the skillet.

4. Sauté the spinach, stirring frequently, until the leaves are wilted and tender, which should take about 3-4 minutes.

5. Season the spinach with salt and pepper to taste. If desired, add a squeeze of lemon juice or a sprinkle of red pepper flakes for an additional flavor boost.

6. Serve the sautéed spinach immediately as a healthy and flavorful side dish.

Nutritional Facts (per serving):

- Calories: 80
- Total Fat: 7g
- Total Carbs: 4g
- Fiber: 2g
- Net Carbs: 2g
- Protein: 2g

***Cooking Tip:** Be careful not to overcook the spinach; it should be bright green and just wilted. You can also add other ingredients like pine nuts, raisins, or a sprinkle of Parmesan cheese for added texture and flavor. Sautéed spinach with garlic is a versatile side that pairs well with a wide range of main dishes, from grilled meats to pasta. This dish is a quick and easy way to include more leafy greens in your diet.*

Recipe 59: Cauliflower Rice Pilaf

Prep Time: 10 mins - Cooking Time: 15 mins - Serves: 4

Ingredients:
1 large head of cauliflower, riced (or 4 cups pre-riced cauliflower)
2 tablespoons olive oil
1 small onion, finely chopped
2 garlic cloves, minced
1/2 cup carrots, diced
1/2 cup celery, diced
1/2 teaspoon ground cumin
1/2 teaspoon dried thyme
Salt and pepper to taste
1/4 cup fresh parsley, chopped
Optional: Chicken or vegetable broth for added flavor, nuts like almonds or pine nuts for crunch

Instructions:
1. If you're using a whole cauliflower, pulse the florets in a food processor until they resemble rice grains. Be careful not to over-process.
2. Heat the olive oil in a large skillet over medium heat. Add the chopped onion and sauté until translucent, about 3-4 minutes.
3. Add the minced garlic, diced carrots, and celery to the skillet. Cook for an additional 3-4 minutes or until the vegetables start to soften.
4. Stir in the riced cauliflower, ground cumin, dried thyme, salt, and pepper. Cook for 5-7 minutes, stirring occasionally, until the cauliflower is tender but not mushy.
5. If using, add a splash of broth to keep the pilaf moist and flavorful.
6. Remove from heat and stir in the chopped parsley. If desired, sprinkle with toasted nuts for added texture and flavor.
7. Serve the cauliflower rice pilaf as a low-carb side dish, perfect for accompanying a variety of main courses.

Nutritional Facts (per serving):
- Calories: 120
- Total Fat: 7g
- Total Carbs: 13g
- Fiber: 4g
- Net Carbs: 9g
- Protein: 3g

Cooking Tip: *You can customize this pilaf by adding different herbs and spices based on your preference. For a Mediterranean twist, include olives, sun-dried tomatoes, and feta cheese. You can also add proteins like cooked chicken, shrimp, or tofu to turn it into a complete meal. Cauliflower rice pilaf is a versatile dish that can adapt to various dietary needs and preferences.*

Recipe 60: Grilled Asparagus with Lemon Butter

Prep Time: 10 mins - Cooking Time: 10 mins - Serves: 4

Ingredients:

1 pound fresh asparagus, trimmed
2 tablespoons olive oil
Salt and pepper to taste
2 tablespoons butter
Zest and juice of 1 lemon
Optional: Grated Parmesan cheese or crushed garlic for extra flavor

Instructions:

1. Preheat your grill to medium-high heat.

2. Toss the asparagus spears with olive oil, salt, and pepper in a bowl, ensuring they are evenly coated.

3. Place the asparagus spears on the grill in a single layer. Grill for about 5-7 minutes, turning occasionally, until they are tender and slightly charred.

4. While the asparagus is grilling, melt the butter in a small saucepan or in the microwave. Stir in the lemon zest and lemon juice. If using, add crushed garlic to the lemon butter for added flavor.

5. Once the asparagus is grilled, transfer it to a serving platter.

6. Drizzle the lemon butter sauce over the grilled asparagus.

7. If desired, sprinkle with grated Parmesan cheese.

8. Serve the grilled asparagus with lemon butter immediately as a delicious and elegant side dish.

Nutritional Facts (per serving):

- Calories: 120
- Total Fat: 10g
- Total Carbs: 5g
- Fiber: 2g
- Net Carbs: 3g
- Protein: 2g

Cooking Tip: *For a smoky flavor, you can add a sprinkle of smoked paprika to the asparagus before grilling. The asparagus can also be cooked in a grill pan over the stove if an outdoor grill is not available. This dish pairs well with grilled meats fish, or can be served as part of a vegetarian meal. For a vegan version, use a plant-based butter alternative.*

Bonus Recipes (with corresponding Chapter as reference)

Chapter 11: Morning Eats. Delicious Breakfast Choices

Recipe 61: Fresh Berry Medley with Greek Yogurt: A straightforward combination of a variety of berries cooked down into a sauce served over creamy Greek yogurt.

Recipe 62: Flavorful Quinoa Breakfast Bowl: A nourishing bowl of quinoa topped with creamy avocado, juicy cherry tomatoes, and a poached egg. Seasoned with herbs for a burst of flavor.

Recipe 63: Spiced Pumpkin Oatmeal: Cozy and comforting oatmeal infused with the flavors of pumpkin puree and a blend of autumn spices. It is topped off with pecans for added texture.

Recipe 64: Cottage. Fresh Fruit Platter: A light and refreshing breakfast option featuring cottage cheese accompanied by an assortment of fruits.

Recipe 65: Smoked Salmon and Creamy Cheese Croissant: A breakfast croissant filled with slices of smoked salmon, luscious cream cheese, and fragrant fresh dill.

Chapter 12: Afternoon Delights. Favorite Lunches

Recipe 66: Zesty Asian Noodle Salad with Peanut Sauce: A refreshing and tangy noodle salad tossed in a peanut dressing combined with vegetables for a satisfying crunch.

Recipe 67: Curried Egg Salad Sandwich Twist: A take on the classic egg salad sandwich infused with curry flavors. Served on grain bread.

Recipe 68: Lentil and Vegetable Soup: This soup is both hearty and healthy, made with lentils, carrots, celery, and tomatoes. It is seasoned with a blend of herbs.

Recipe 69: Chickpea and Avocado Wrap: Enjoy a wrap filled with chickpeas, sliced avocado, and mixed greens. It is all brought together with a lemon tahini sauce.

Recipe 70: Quiche with Spinach and Mushrooms: Treat yourself to a quiche packed with spinach, mushrooms, and cheese. It's the choice for lunch.

Chapter 13: The Heart of Dining. Main Course Creations

Recipe 71: Herb-Crusted Rack of Lamb: Indulge in the succulent flavors of this rack of lamb coated in a herb crust. Roasted to perfection. Served alongside a red wine reduction.

Recipe 72: Vegetarian Stuffed Bell Peppers: Delight in bell peppers stuffed generously with a mixture of quinoa, black beans, corn, and spices. It is topped off with melted cheese for a touch of goodness.

Recipe 73: Coconut Shrimp Curry: Experience the creamy yet delight of this curry featuring tender shrimp cooked in coconut milk infused with aromatic spices.

Recipe 74: Eggplant Rollatini: Savor the layers of sliced eggplant rolled up with ricotta cheese and spinach. Baked to perfection in marinara sauce. Topped off generously with mozzarella.

Recipe 75: Beef Bourguignon: A timeless French stew that combines succulent beef chunks, earthy mushrooms, carrots, and onions in a sauce infused with the flavors of wine.

Chapter 14: Indulgent Yet Healthy. Snacks & Desserts

Recipe 76: Energy Packed Matcha Green Tea Bites: bites bursting with nutrients created using powder, oats, and a medley of nuts. Perfect for a quick and refreshing energy boost.

Recipe 77: Honey Glazed Baked Peaches, with Almonds: Succulent peaches gently baked to perfection, drizzled with honey, and adorned with a sprinkling of almonds. An effortless yet refined dessert.

Recipe 78: Decadent Flourless Chocolate Cake: An indulgent chocolate cake that's completely devoid of flour, making it an ideal treat for those who follow a gluten-free lifestyle.

Recipe 79: Assorted Nut and Seed Trail Mix: A trail mix brimming with an array of nuts and seeds delicately seasoned and lightly roasted to enhance flavors.

Recipe 80: Delicate Raspberry Coconut Bars: A confection featuring a coconut-infused base topped with raspberries delicately sweetened for the perfect balance of flavors.

Chapter 15: Harmonizing Complements. Side Dishes

Recipe 81: Roasted Cauliflower Infused with Garlic and Parmesan; Tender cauliflower florets expertly roasted to achieve a crispy texture generously seasoned with Parmesan cheese. A mouthwatering side dish that will leave you craving more.

Recipe 82: Fragrant Wild Rice Pilaf Infused with Herbs: This is a savory dish featuring aromatic wild rice enhanced with a blend of fresh herbs. This recipe offers a delightful combination of textures and flavors, perfect as a wholesome side or a light main course.

Here are a few delicious side dishes you can try;

Recipe 83: Zucchini and Corn Fritters: These fritters are crispy and made with zucchini and corn. They're seasoned with herbs. Served alongside a creamy yogurt dip.

Recipe 84: Maple Glazed Carrots: Take your carrots to the next level by roasting them with a maple syrup glaze. This adds a touch of elegance to any meal.

Recipe 85: Grilled Vegetable Platter: Create a platter of grilled vegetables, including bell peppers, zucchini, and eggplant. These veggies are beautifully seasoned with herbs for added flavor.

Enjoy these dishes. Elevate your meals!

Recipe 61: Mixed Berry Compote with Greek Yogurt

Prep Time: 5 mins - Cooking Time: 10 mins - Serves: 4

Ingredients:

2 cups mixed berries (such as strawberries, blueberries, raspberries, and blackberries)
1/4 cup sugar or honey (adjust to taste)
1 teaspoon lemon juice
1/2 teaspoon vanilla extract
2 cups Greek yogurt

Instructions:

1. In a saucepan, combine the mixed berries, sugar or honey, and lemon juice. Cook over medium heat.

2. As the berries warm up and release their juices, stir gently and occasionally, mashing some of the berries with the back of the spoon for a thicker compote.

3. Simmer the mixture for about 8-10 minutes or until it thickens slightly. Be careful not to overcook; the berries should still retain some of their shape.

4. Remove from heat and stir in the vanilla extract.

5. Let the compote cool down a bit. It can be served warm or chilled, depending on your preference.

6. To serve, spoon the Greek yogurt into bowls and top with the mixed berry compote.

7. Serve immediately as a refreshing and healthy dessert or breakfast option.

Nutritional Facts (per serving):

- Calories: 180
- Total Fat: 4g
- Total Carbs: 28g
- Fiber: 2g
- Net Carbs: 26g
- Protein: 10g

Cooking Tip: You can adjust the sweetness of the compote to your liking by adding more or less sugar or honey. For a more complex flavor, you can add a pinch of cinnamon or nutmeg to the compote while cooking. This recipe is very versatile – you can use frozen berries instead of fresh ones, and you can also experiment with different types of fruit. The compote can be stored in the refrigerator for up to a week and can be used as a topping for pancakes, waffles, or oatmeal.

Recipe 62: Savory Breakfast Quinoa Bowl

Prep Time: 10 mins - Cooking Time: 20 mins - Serves: 2

Ingredients:
1 cup quinoa, rinsed
2 cups water or vegetable broth
1 ripe avocado, sliced
1/2 cup cherry tomatoes, halved
2 eggs
1 tablespoon white vinegar (for poaching eggs)
Salt and pepper to taste
Fresh herbs (such as parsley, chives, or cilantro), chopped
Optional: Red pepper flakes, lemon juice, or a drizzle of olive oil for extra flavor

Instructions:
1. In a medium saucepan, bring the water or broth to a boil. Add the rinsed quinoa, reduce heat to low, cover, and simmer for about 15 minutes, or until all the liquid is absorbed and the quinoa is fluffy.
2. While the quinoa is cooking, poach the eggs. Bring a pot of water to a gentle simmer and add the white vinegar. Crack each egg into a small bowl and gently slide it into the simmering water. Cook for about 3-4 minutes for a soft yolk or longer for a firmer yolk. Remove the eggs with a slotted spoon and set aside on a paper towel.
3. Assemble the breakfast bowls by dividing the cooked quinoa into two servings. Top each bowl with sliced avocado, cherry tomatoes, and a poached egg.
4. Season with salt, pepper, and fresh herbs. If desired, add red pepper flakes, a squeeze of lemon juice, or a drizzle of olive oil for extra flavor.
5. Serve the savory breakfast quinoa bowls immediately, offering a wholesome and satisfying start to the day.

Nutritional Facts (per serving):
- Calories: 400
- Total Fat: 15g
- Total Carbs: 50g
- Fiber: 8g
- Net Carbs: 42g
- Protein: 16g

Cooking Tip: You can customize the quinoa bowls with additional toppings like sautéed spinach, mushrooms, or crumbled feta cheese. For a vegan version, substitute the egg with a tofu scramble or a dollop of hummus. This dish is not only great for breakfast but can also serve as a healthy lunch option. The quinoa can be cooked in advance and stored in the refrigerator for quick assembly in the morning.

Recipe 63: Pumpkin Spice Oatmeal

Prep Time: 5 mins - Cooking Time: 10 mins - Serves: 2

Ingredients:
1 cup rolled oats
2 cups milk or water (or a combination of both)
1/2 cup pumpkin puree
1/4 cup brown sugar or maple syrup (adjust to taste)
1 teaspoon ground cinnamon
1/2 teaspoon ground nutmeg
1/4 teaspoon ground ginger
1/4 teaspoon ground cloves
Pinch of salt
1/4 cup pecans, chopped
Optional: Additional toppings like sliced bananas, a dollop of Greek yogurt, or a drizzle of honey

Instructions:
1. In a medium saucepan, bring the milk or water to a boil. Add the rolled oats and a pinch of salt, then reduce the heat to a simmer.
2. Stir in the pumpkin puree, brown sugar or maple syrup, cinnamon, nutmeg, ginger, and cloves. Mix well until everything is fully incorporated.
3. Cook the oatmeal for about 5-7 minutes or until it reaches your desired consistency, stirring occasionally.
4. Once the oatmeal is cooked, remove it from heat and let it sit for a couple of minutes to thicken.
5. Serve the pumpkin spice oatmeal in bowls, topped with chopped pecans. If desired, add additional toppings like sliced bananas, Greek yogurt, or a drizzle of honey.
6. Enjoy the warm and comforting flavors of this autumn-inspired oatmeal.

Nutritional Facts (per serving):
- Calories: 320
- Total Fat: 10g
- Total Carbs: 50g
- Fiber: 7g
- Net Carbs: 43g
- Protein: 10g

Cooking Tip: For a creamier texture, use milk or a mix of milk and water. You can also make this oatmeal in the microwave by combining all ingredients in a microwave-safe bowl and cooking for 2-3 minutes, stirring halfway through. The recipe can be easily doubled or adjusted for more servings. Feel free to customize the spice levels to your preference. This oatmeal can also be made in advance and reheated, adding a little extra milk or water to loosen it up if needed.

Recipe 64: Cottage Cheese and Fruit Plate

Prep Time: 5 mins - No Cooking - Serves: 2

Ingredients:

1 cup cottage cheese
1/2 cup fresh strawberries, sliced
1/2 cup fresh blueberries
1/2 cup fresh pineapple, diced
1 kiwi, sliced
Optional: Honey or maple syrup for drizzling, nuts or seeds for added texture, fresh mint for garnish

Instructions:

1. Divide the cottage cheese between two plates, placing it as a base.

2. Arrange the sliced strawberries, blueberries, diced pineapple, and kiwi slices around the cottage cheese on each plate.

3. If desired, drizzle a little honey or maple syrup over the cottage cheese and fruit for added sweetness.

4. Optionally, sprinkle some nuts or seeds (such as almonds, chia seeds, or sunflower seeds) over the plates for added crunch and nutrition.

5. Garnish with fresh mint leaves for a refreshing touch.

6. Serve the cottage cheese and fruit plates immediately as a light and refreshing breakfast or snack option.

Nutritional Facts (per serving):

- Calories: 200
- Total Fat: 3g
- Total Carbs: 30g
- Fiber: 4g
- Net Carbs: 26g
- Protein: 15g

Cooking Tip: *This dish is highly customizable based on your personal preferences and the seasonal availability of fruits. You can experiment with different fruit combinations, such as mixed berries, sliced peaches, or mango. For a savory twist, you can top the cottage cheese with sliced tomatoes, cucumber, and a sprinkle of salt and pepper. Cottage cheese is a great source of protein and can be a satisfying yet light meal option.*

Recipe 65: Smoked Salmon and Cream Cheese Croissant

Prep Time: 10 mins - No Cooking - Serves: 2

Ingredients:

2 croissants, sliced in half
4 ounces smoked salmon
1/4 cup cream cheese, softened
Fresh dill, chopped
1/4 red onion, thinly sliced
Optional: Capers lemon wedges for serving

Instructions:

1. Spread a generous layer of cream cheese on each half of the croissants.

2. Place slices of smoked salmon over the bottom halves of the croissants.

3. Sprinkle chopped fresh dill and add a few slices of red onion on top of the salmon.

4. If using, add a few capers for an extra burst of flavor.

5. Cover with the top halves of the croissants.

6. Serve the smoked salmon and cream cheese croissants immediately, accompanied by lemon wedges if desired.

Nutritional Facts (per serving):

- Calories: 400
- Total Fat: 22g
- Total Carbs: 29g
- Fiber: 2g
- Net Carbs: 27g
- Protein: 18g

Cooking Tip: *For a healthier version, you can use whole wheat or multigrain croissants. Alternatively, bagels can be used in place of croissants. For a different flavor profile, you can add a pinch of black pepper, a squeeze of lemon juice, or a spread of avocado to the croissants. This dish is perfect for a luxurious weekend breakfast or brunch.*

Recipe 66: Asian Noodle Salad with Peanut Dressing

Prep Time: 20 mins - No Cooking (if using pre-cooked noodles) - Serves: 4

Ingredients:
For the Salad:
8 ounces Asian noodles (such as soba, rice noodles, or linguine)
1 red bell pepper, thinly sliced
1 carrot, julienned or shredded
1 cucumber, julienned or thinly sliced
1/2 cup red cabbage, shredded
1/4 cup green onions, chopped
1/4 cup fresh cilantro, chopped
Optional: Crushed peanuts, sesame seeds, or lime wedges for garnish

For the Peanut Dressing:
1/4 cup peanut butter, smooth or crunchy
2 tablespoons soy sauce
1 tablespoon rice vinegar or lime juice
1 tablespoon honey or maple syrup
1 teaspoon sesame oil
1 garlic clove, minced
1 teaspoon grated ginger
1-2 tablespoons water (or more to thin the dressing)

Instructions:
1. Cook the noodles according to the package instructions. Rinse under cold water and drain.
2. In a large bowl, combine the cooked noodles, red bell pepper, carrot, cucumber, red cabbage, green onions, and cilantro.
3. To make the peanut dressing, whisk together the peanut butter, soy sauce, rice vinegar or lime juice, honey or maple syrup, sesame oil, minced garlic, and grated ginger in a bowl. Gradually add water until the dressing reaches a pourable consistency.
4. Pour the peanut dressing over the noodle salad and toss well to coat all the ingredients.
5. Serve the Asian noodle salad garnished with crushed peanuts, sesame seeds, or lime wedges if desired.

Nutritional Facts (per serving):
- Calories: 350
- Total Fat: 12g
- Total Carbs: 52g
- Fiber: 4g
- Net Carbs: 48g
- Protein: 12g

Cooking Tip: *You can add cooked chicken, shrimp, or tofu for extra protein. The salad can be customized with other vegetables like snap peas, bell peppers, or edamame. For a spicier dressing, add a squirt of sriracha or a pinch of red pepper flakes. This noodle salad is great for picnics or as a make-ahead meal, as the flavors develop more over time.*

Recipe 67: Curried Egg Salad Sandwich

Prep Time: 15 mins - Cooking Time: 10 mins (for eggs) - Serves: 2

Ingredients:
4 large eggs
1/4 cup mayonnaise
1 teaspoon curry powder
1/2 teaspoon Dijon mustard
Salt and pepper to taste
1/4 cup celery, finely chopped
2 tablespoons red onion, finely chopped
4 slices whole grain bread
Optional: Lettuce leaves, sliced tomatoes, or cucumber slices for added crunch and freshness

Instructions:
1. Place the eggs in a saucepan and cover them with cold water. Bring the water to a boil, then reduce the heat and simmer for 10 minutes.
2. Drain the hot water and immediately run cold water over the eggs to cool them quickly. Peel the eggs once they are cool enough to handle.
3. In a bowl, mash the boiled eggs with a fork or potato masher.
4. Add the mayonnaise, curry powder, Dijon mustard, salt, and pepper to the mashed eggs. Stir until well combined.
5. Mix in the chopped celery and red onion.
6. Toast the whole grain bread slices.
7. Spread a generous amount of the curried egg salad onto two slices of the toasted bread. If desired, add lettuce leaves, sliced tomatoes, or cucumber slices.
8. Top with the remaining slices of bread.
9. Cut the sandwiches in half and serve immediately.

Nutritional Facts (per sandwich):
- Calories: 400
- Total Fat: 22g
- Total Carbs: 30g
- Fiber: 5g
- Net Carbs: 25g
- Protein: 20g

Cooking Tip: *For a healthier version, you can substitute mayonnaise with Greek yogurt or a combination of both. Adjust the amount of curry powder to suit your taste preferences. This curried egg salad can also be served on a bed of greens for a low-carb option. The salad can be made in advance and stored in the refrigerator for quick assembly.*

Recipe 68: Lentil and Vegetable Soup

Prep Time: 15 mins - Cooking Time: 45 mins - Serves: 4-6

Ingredients:
1 cup dried lentils, rinsed and drained
2 tablespoons olive oil
1 onion, chopped
2 carrots, peeled and diced
2 celery stalks, diced
3 garlic cloves, minced
1 can (14.5 ounces) diced tomatoes with their juice
6 cups vegetable broth or water
1 teaspoon dried thyme
1 teaspoon dried basil
Salt and pepper to taste
Optional: Spinach or kale, chopped parsley, and lemon juice for serving

Instructions:
1. In a large pot, heat the olive oil over medium heat. Add the chopped onion, carrots, and celery. Sauté until the vegetables are softened, about 5 minutes.
2. Add the minced garlic and cook for another minute until fragrant.
3. Stir in the diced tomatoes, dried lentils, vegetable broth or water, thyme, and basil. Bring the mixture to a boil.
4. Reduce the heat to low, cover, and simmer for about 35-40 minutes or until the lentils are tender.
5. Season the soup with salt and pepper to taste. If using, add the chopped spinach or kale towards the end of the cooking time and cook until wilted.
6. Serve the lentil and vegetable soup hot, garnished with chopped parsley and a squeeze of lemon juice if desired.

Nutritional Facts (per serving):
- Calories: 220
- Total Fat: 5g
- Total Carbs: 33g
- Fiber: 15g
- Net Carbs: 18g
- Protein: 12g

Cooking Tip: *You can use any lentils for this recipe, but brown or green lentils hold their shape well during cooking. For a richer flavor, you can sauté the vegetables in a bit of butter along with the olive oil. This soup is versatile, so feel free to add other vegetables like potatoes, bell peppers, or zucchini. It can be stored in the refrigerator for up to 4 days or frozen for longer storage. The soup thickens as it cools, so you may need to add more broth or water when reheating.*

Recipe 69: Chickpea and Avocado Wrap

Prep Time: 15 mins - No Cooking - Serves: 2

Ingredients:

1 can (15 ounces) chickpeas, drained and rinsed
1 ripe avocado, sliced
2 large tortillas or wraps
1 cup mixed greens (like spinach, arugula, or lettuce)
Salt and pepper to taste

For the Lemon-Tahini Sauce:

3 tablespoons tahini
2 tablespoons lemon juice
1 garlic clove, minced
2-3 tablespoons water (to thin the sauce)
Salt to taste

Instructions:

1. In a bowl, mash the chickpeas with a fork or potato masher until they are broken down but still have some texture.
2. Prepare the lemon-tahini sauce by whisking together tahini, lemon juice, minced garlic, and enough water to reach a pourable consistency. Season with salt to taste.
3. Lay out the tortillas or wraps and spread a layer of the smashed chickpeas on each.
4. Place slices of avocado on top of the chickpeas.
5. Add a handful of mixed greens to each wrap.
6. Drizzle the lemon-tahini sauce over the greens.
7. Season with salt and pepper.
8. Carefully roll up the wraps, tucking in the sides as you go.
9. Slice the wraps in half and serve immediately.

Nutritional Facts (per serving):

- Calories: 450
- Total Fat: 20g
- Total Carbs: 55g
- Fiber: 15g
- Net Carbs: 40g
- Protein: 15g

***Cooking Tip:** For added flavor, you can include ingredients like sliced cucumbers, bell peppers, or sun-dried tomatoes in the wrap. If you like it spicy, add a few dashes of hot sauce or sprinkle some chili flakes into the chickpea mixture. This wrap is great for a quick lunch and can be easily customized to suit your taste preferences. If preparing in advance, add the avocado and sauce just before serving to keep the wrap fresh.*

Recipe 70: Quiche with Spinach and Mushrooms

Prep Time: 20 mins - Cooking Time: 35-40 mins - Serves: 6

Ingredients:

1 pie crust (store-bought or homemade)
2 tablespoons olive oil
1 onion, finely chopped
2 cups mushrooms, sliced
2 cups spinach, washed and roughly chopped
4 large eggs
1 cup heavy cream or milk
1 cup grated cheese (such as Gruyère, Swiss, or cheddar)
Salt and pepper to taste
Optional: Nutmeg, garlic, or herbs like thyme for extra flavor

Instructions:

1. Preheat the oven to 375°F (190°C). Place the pie crust in a 9-inch quiche or tart pan, trimming any excess dough. Prick the bottom with a fork and set aside.
2. In a skillet, heat the olive oil over medium heat. Add the chopped onion and sauté until translucent, about 5 minutes.
3. Add the sliced mushrooms and cook until they release their moisture and begin to brown.
4. Stir in the spinach and cook until just wilted. Season with salt, pepper, and any additional spices or herbs if using. Remove from heat and let the mixture cool slightly.
5. In a bowl, whisk together the eggs and heavy cream (or milk). Stir in the grated cheese.
6. Spread the spinach and mushroom mixture evenly over the crust. Pour the egg and cheese mixture on top.
7. Bake in the preheated oven for 35-40 minutes or until the quiche is set and the crust is golden brown.
8. Remove from the oven and let it cool for a few minutes before slicing.
9. Serve the quiche warm or at room temperature.

Nutritional Facts (per serving):
- Calories: 380
- Total Fat: 28g
- Total Carbs: 20g
- Fiber: 2g
- Net Carbs: 18g
- Protein: 15g

Cooking Tip: You can blind-bake the crust for 10 minutes before adding the filling to prevent a soggy bottom. Feel free to experiment with different vegetables and cheeses according to your preference. A quiche can be made ahead and either served at room temperature or reheated. It's also a great dish for brunches, parties, or as a make-ahead meal.

Recipe 71: Herb-Crusted Rack of Lamb

Prep Time: 20 mins - Cooking Time: 25 mins - Serves: 4

Ingredients:
For the Lamb:
1 rack of lamb (about 8 ribs)
2 tablespoons olive oil
Salt and pepper to taste
1/4 cup fresh bread crumbs
2 tablespoons fresh rosemary, finely chopped
2 tablespoons fresh thyme, finely chopped
2 garlic cloves, minced
2 tablespoons Dijon mustard

For the Red Wine Reduction:
1 cup red wine
1/2 cup chicken or beef broth
1 shallot, minced
1 sprig of thyme
Salt and pepper to taste
Optional: 1 tablespoon butter

Instructions:
1. Preheat the oven to 400°F (200°C).
2. Season the rack of lamb with salt and pepper. Heat the olive oil in a large ovenproof skillet over high heat. Sear the lamb on all sides until golden brown, about 2-3 minutes per side. Remove from heat.
3. In a bowl, mix together the bread crumbs, chopped rosemary, thyme, and minced garlic.
4. Brush the Dijon mustard over the lamb, then press the herb and breadcrumb mixture onto the meat, coating it evenly.
5. Place the skillet with the lamb in the preheated oven and roast for about 20-25 minutes for medium-rare or until it reaches your desired level of doneness.
6. While the lamb is roasting, make the red wine reduction. In a saucepan, combine the red wine, broth, minced shallot, and thyme sprig. Bring to a simmer and cook until the sauce is reduced by half. Season with salt and pepper. If using, whisk in the butter at the end for a richer sauce.
7. Remove the lamb from the oven and let it rest for 10 minutes before slicing between the ribs.
8. Serve the herb-crusted rack of lamb with the red wine reduction drizzled over the top.

Nutritional Facts (per serving):
- Calories: 450
- Total Fat: 25g
- Total Carbs: 8g
- Fiber: 1g
- Net Carbs: 7g
- Protein: 40g

***Cooking Tip:** Letting the lamb rest before slicing ensures the juices redistribute for a more tender and flavorful meat. You can adjust the herbs in the crust according to your preferences or add ingredients like Parmesan cheese for extra flavor. The red wine reduction can be made in advance and reheated when serving*

Recipe 72: Vegetarian Stuffed Bell Peppers

Prep Time: 20 mins - Cooking Time: 30 mins - Serves: 4

Ingredients:
4 large bell peppers, any color, tops cut off and seeds removed
1 cup quinoa, cooked
1 can (15 ounces) black beans, drained and rinsed
1 cup corn (fresh, canned, or frozen)
1/2 cup red onion, finely chopped
2 garlic cloves, minced
1 teaspoon ground cumin
1/2 teaspoon chili powder
1/2 teaspoon smoked paprika
Salt and pepper to taste
1 cup shredded cheese (such as cheddar or Monterey Jack)
Optional: Fresh cilantro, lime wedges, and sour cream for serving

Instructions:
1. Preheat the oven to 375°F (190°C).
2. In a large bowl, combine the cooked quinoa, black beans, corn, red onion, minced garlic, cumin, chili powder, smoked paprika, salt, and pepper. Mix well.
3. Stuff each bell pepper with the quinoa mixture, pressing down gently to fill them completely.
4. Place the stuffed peppers upright in a baking dish. Add a little water to the bottom of the dish (about 1/4 inch) to help steam the peppers.
5. Cover the dish with aluminum foil and bake in the preheated oven for 25 minutes.
6. Remove the foil, top each pepper with shredded cheese, and bake for an additional 5 minutes or until the cheese is melted and bubbly.
7. Serve the vegetarian stuffed bell peppers garnished with fresh cilantro, lime wedges, and a dollop of sour cream if desired.

Nutritional Facts (per serving):
- Calories: 350
- Total Fat: 12g
- Total Carbs: 45g
- Fiber: 10g
- Net Carbs: 35g
- Protein: 18g

Cooking Tip: You can customize the filling by adding other vegetables like diced tomatoes or zucchini. For a vegan version, use a plant-based cheese or omit the cheese topping. These stuffed peppers are great for meal prep as they reheat well and can be stored in the refrigerator for a few days. The recipe can also be easily doubled to serve more people or to have leftovers.

Recipe 73: Coconut Shrimp Curry

Prep Time: 15 mins - Cooking Time: 25 mins - Serves: 4

Ingredients:
1 pound large shrimp, peeled and deveined
2 tablespoons vegetable oil
1 onion, finely chopped
3 garlic cloves, minced
1 tablespoon ginger, grated
1 red bell pepper, sliced
1 can (14 ounces) coconut milk
2 tablespoons tomato paste
1 tablespoon curry powder
1/2 teaspoon ground turmeric
1/2 teaspoon chili powder (adjust to taste)
Salt to taste
Fresh cilantro, chopped for garnish
Optional: Lime wedges for serving

Instructions:
1. In a large skillet or saucepan, heat the vegetable oil over medium heat. Add the chopped onion and sauté until translucent, about 5 minutes.
2. Add the minced garlic and grated ginger, cooking for another minute until fragrant.
3. Stir in the red bell pepper and cook for 2-3 minutes until slightly softened.
4. Add the coconut milk, tomato paste, curry powder, turmeric, chili powder, and salt. Stir well to combine all the ingredients.
5. Bring the mixture to a simmer and cook for 10 minutes, allowing the flavors to meld together.
6. Add the shrimp to the curry and cook for 5-7 minutes, or until the shrimp are pink and cooked through.
7. Adjust the seasoning, adding more salt or chili powder if needed.
8. Garnish with chopped cilantro and serve with lime wedges if desired.
9. Serve the coconut shrimp curry hot, over rice, or with naan bread.

Nutritional Facts (per serving):
- Calories: 350
- Total Fat: 22g
- Total Carbs: 12g
- Fiber: 2g
- Net Carbs: 10g
- Protein: 25g

Cooking Tip: For a thicker curry, you can add a teaspoon of cornstarch dissolved in water towards the end of cooking. You can also include vegetables like spinach, zucchini, or tomatoes. For a vegetarian version, substitute the shrimp with tofu or chickpeas. This dish can be made spicier by adding more chili powder or by using fresh chili peppers. The curry can be stored in the refrigerator for up to 3 days and reheated, making it a great option for meal prep.

Recipe 74: Eggplant Rollatini

Prep Time: 30 mins - Cooking Time: 30 mins - Serves: 4-6

Ingredients:
2 large eggplants, sliced lengthwise into 1/4-inch thick slices
Salt
2 tablespoons olive oil
1 cup ricotta cheese
1 cup spinach, cooked and drained
1 egg
1/2 cup grated Parmesan cheese
1 teaspoon garlic powder
1/2 teaspoon dried basil
1/2 teaspoon dried oregano
Pepper to taste
2 cups marinara sauce
1 cup shredded mozzarella cheese

Instructions:
1. Preheat the oven to 375°F (190°C).
2. Sprinkle salt on the eggplant slices and set them aside for 10-15 minutes to draw out moisture. Pat them dry with paper towels.
3. Brush each eggplant slice with olive oil and place them on a baking sheet. Bake for 8-10 minutes until just tender.
4. In a bowl, mix together the ricotta cheese, spinach, egg, Parmesan cheese, garlic powder, basil, oregano, salt, and pepper.
5. Spread a thin layer of marinara sauce on the bottom of a baking dish.
6. Place a spoonful of the ricotta-spinach mixture on one end of each eggplant slice and roll up tightly.
7. Place the eggplant rolls seam-side down in the prepared baking dish.
8. Pour the remaining marinara sauce over the eggplant rolls.
9. Sprinkle with shredded mozzarella cheese.
10. Bake for 20-25 minutes or until the cheese is melted and bubbly.
11. Serve the eggplant rollatini hot, garnished with additional Parmesan cheese or fresh basil if desired.

Nutritional Facts (per serving):
- Calories: 320
- Total Fat: 18g
- Total Carbs: 22g
- Fiber: 6g
- Net Carbs: 16g
- Protein: 18g

Cooking Tip: *For a richer flavor, you can add a layer of sautéed onions or mushrooms to the ricotta-spinach mixture. To make this dish lighter, you can use part-skim ricotta and mozzarella cheese. Eggplant rollatini can be made ahead and reheated, making it a great option for entertaining or meal prep. If you prefer a vegetarian dish, ensure the marinara sauce is free of meat products.*

Recipe 75: Beef Bourguignon

Prep Time: 20 mins - Cooking Time: 2-3 hrs - Serves: 6

Ingredients:

2 pounds beef chuck, cut into 2-inch cubes
Salt and freshly ground black pepper to taste
3 tablespoons olive oil
4 slices bacon, chopped
1 large onion, chopped
3 carrots, sliced into 1-inch pieces
3 garlic cloves, minced
1 bottle (750 ml) dry red wine, such as Burgundy or Pinot Noir
2 cups beef stock
2 tablespoons tomato paste
1 teaspoon fresh thyme leaves or 1/2 teaspoon dried thyme
1 bay leaf
1 pound mushrooms, quartered
2 tablespoons butter
2 tablespoons all-purpose flour
Optional: Chopped parsley for garnish

Instructions:

1. Pat the beef dry with paper towels and season with salt and pepper. In a large Dutch oven or heavy-bottomed pot, heat 1 tablespoon of olive oil over medium-high heat. Brown the beef in batches, ensuring the pan is not overcrowded, and set aside.
2. In the same pot, cook the bacon until crisp. Remove the bacon and set aside, leaving the fat in the pot.
3. Reduce the heat to medium. Add the onions and carrots, and cook until softened about 5 minutes. Add the garlic and cook for another minute.
4. Pour in the wine, scraping up any browned bits from the bottom of the pot. Add the beef stock, tomato paste, thyme, bay leaf, and the browned beef and bacon. Bring to a simmer.
5. Cover and simmer gently for about 2 hours or until the beef is very tender.
6. In a separate skillet, heat the remaining 2 tablespoons of olive oil. Add the mushrooms and cook until browned.
7. In a small bowl, mash together the butter and flour to make a paste (beurre manié).
8. Stir the cooked mushrooms and the beurre manié into the stew. Simmer for another 10-15 minutes or until the sauce thickens slightly.
9. Discard the bay leaf and adjust the seasoning with salt and pepper.
10. Serve the beef bourguignon hot, garnished with chopped parsley if desired.

Nutritional Facts (per serving):

- Calories: 550
- Total Fat: 30g
- Total Carbs: 20g
- Fiber: 2g
- Net Carbs: 18g
- Protein: 40g

Cooking Tip: Beef bourguignon tastes even better the next day, as the flavors have more time to meld together. It can be served over mashed potatoes, noodles, or with crusty bread. For a gluten-free version, you can thicken the stew with cornstarch dissolved in a little cold water instead of using flour.

Recipe 76: Matcha Green Tea Energy Bites

Prep Time: 15 mins - No Cooking - Makes: 12-15 bites

Ingredients:

1 cup rolled oats

1/2 cup nut butter (almond, peanut, or cashew)

1/4 cup honey or maple syrup

2 tablespoons chia seeds

2 tablespoons flaxseed meal

2 teaspoons matcha green tea powder

1/2 cup nuts (almonds, walnuts, or pecans), finely chopped

Optional: Shredded coconut, mini chocolate chips, or dried fruit for added flavor

Instructions:

1. In a large bowl, mix together the rolled oats, nut butter, honey or maple syrup, chia seeds, flaxseed meal, and matcha powder. Stir until well combined.

2. Add the finely chopped nuts to the mixture and stir to distribute evenly.

3. Using your hands, roll the mixture into small balls about 1 inch in diameter. If the mixture is too sticky, refrigerate it for about 15-20 minutes before rolling.

4. Optionally, roll the energy bites in shredded coconut, mini chocolate chips, or dried fruit for an extra layer of flavor and texture.

5. Place the matcha green tea energy bites on a plate or tray and refrigerate for at least 30 minutes to firm up.

6. Store the energy bites in an airtight container in the refrigerator.

Nutritional Facts (per bite):

- Calories: 100

- Total Fat: 6g

- Total Carbs: 10g

- Fiber: 2g

- Net Carbs: 8g

- Protein: 3g

Cooking Tip*: Matcha powder can vary in intensity, so you may want to adjust the quantity to suit your taste. These energy bites are a convenient snack for on-the-go. They can be customized according to your dietary preferences and the ingredients you have on hand. For a vegan option, ensure that the maple syrup is used as a sweetener. The energy bites can also be frozen for longer storage.*

Recipe 77: Baked Peaches with Honey and Almonds

Prep Time: 10 mins - Cooking Time: 15-20 mins - Serves: 4

Ingredients:

4 ripe peaches, halved and pitted

4 tablespoons honey

1/2 cup sliced almonds

Optional: A pinch of ground cinnamon or nutmeg

Optional: Vanilla ice cream or Greek yogurt for serving

Instructions:

1. Preheat the oven to 375°F (190°C).

2. Arrange the peach halves, cut side up, in a baking dish.

3. Drizzle each peach half with honey. If using, sprinkle a pinch of ground cinnamon or nutmeg over the peaches for added flavor.

4. Scatter the sliced almonds evenly over the peaches.

5. Bake in the preheated oven for 15-20 minutes or until the peaches are tender and the almonds are lightly toasted.

6. Remove from the oven and let cool slightly.

7. Serve the baked peaches warm, as is, or with a scoop of vanilla ice cream or a dollop of Greek yogurt for an added indulgence.

Nutritional Facts (per serving):

- Calories: 180

- Total Fat: 7g

- Total Carbs: 29g

- Fiber: 3g

- Net Carbs: 26g

- Protein: 4g

Cooking Tip: *Choose peaches that are ripe but still firm enough to hold their shape when baked. The almonds add a delightful crunch, but you can substitute them with other nuts like pecans or walnuts. For a vegan option, use maple syrup or agave syrup instead of honey. This dessert is not only delicious but also quick and easy to prepare, making it perfect for entertaining or a special treat. The natural sweetness of the peaches is enhanced by the baking process, creating a delightful and healthy dessert.*

Recipe 78: Flourless Chocolate Cake

Prep Time: 20 mins - Cooking Time: 25-30 mins - Serves: 8-10

Ingredients:
8 ounces of high-quality dark chocolate, chopped
1/2 cup (1 stick) unsalted butter, plus extra for greasing
1 cup granulated sugar
1/2 cup unsweetened cocoa powder, plus extra for dusting
4 large eggs
1 teaspoon vanilla extract
A pinch of salt

Instructions:
1. Preheat the oven to 350°F (175°C). Grease an 8-inch round cake pan and line the bottom with parchment paper. Lightly dust the sides of the pan with cocoa powder.
2. In a double boiler or a heatproof bowl set over a pot of simmering water, melt the chopped dark chocolate and butter together, stirring until smooth. Remove from heat.
3. In a large bowl, mix together the granulated sugar and cocoa powder. Gradually whisk in the melted chocolate mixture until well combined.
4. Beat in the eggs, one at a time, ensuring each is fully incorporated before adding the next. Stir in the vanilla extract and a pinch of salt.
5. Pour the batter into the prepared cake pan, smoothing the top with a spatula.
6. Bake in the preheated oven for 25-30 minutes, or until the cake is set and a toothpick inserted into the center comes out with moist crumbs.
7. Remove the cake from the oven and let it cool in the pan for about 10 minutes, then invert onto a wire rack to cool completely.
8. Once cooled, dust the top of the cake with additional cocoa powder or decorate as desired.
9. Serve slices of the flourless chocolate cake with whipped cream, fresh berries, or a drizzle of chocolate sauce if desired.

Nutritional Facts (per serving):
- Calories: 320
- Total Fat: 20g
- Total Carbs: 30g
- Fiber: 3g
- Net Carbs: 27g
- Protein: 5g

***Cooking Tip:** Ensure that all ingredients, particularly the eggs and butter, are at room temperature before starting. For a richer flavor, you can add a splash of espresso or your favorite liqueur to the chocolate mixture. This cake is very rich and dense, so smaller servings are recommended. It can be stored in an airtight container for up to 3 days. For those sensitive to caffeine, be mindful of the chocolate content, especially if serving in the evening.*

Recipe 79 - Mixed Nut and Seed Trail Mix

Prep Time: 10 mins - Cooking Time: 20 mins - Serves: 8

Ingredients:
1 cup almonds, raw
1 cup walnuts, raw
1 cup cashews, raw
1/2 cup pumpkin seeds, raw
1/2 cup sunflower seeds, raw
1/4 cup sesame seeds
2 tablespoons chia seeds
1 tablespoon flaxseeds
1 teaspoon sea salt
1/2 teaspoon black pepper, freshly ground
1/2 teaspoon paprika
1 tablespoon olive oil
Optional: 1/2 cup dried cranberries or raisins

Instructions:
1. Preheat your oven to 350°F (175°C). Line a baking tray with parchment paper.
2. In a large bowl, combine almonds, walnuts, cashews, pumpkin seeds, and sunflower seeds. Toss to mix evenly.
3. In a small bowl, mix together sea salt, black pepper, and paprika.
4. Drizzle olive oil over the nuts and seeds, then sprinkle the mixed seasonings over them. Toss to coat everything evenly.
5. Spread the nut and seed mixture in a single layer on the prepared baking tray.
6. Bake in the preheated oven for about 20 minutes or until the nuts and seeds are lightly toasted, stirring halfway through to ensure even roasting.
7. Remove from the oven and let the trail mix cool completely on the tray.
8. Once cooled, add in the sesame seeds, chia seeds, flaxseeds, and optional dried cranberries or raisins. Toss to combine.
9. Store the trail mix in an airtight container at room temperature for up to 2 weeks.

Nutritional Facts (per serving):
- Calories: 210
- Total Fat: 18g
- Saturated Fat: 2g
- Cholesterol: 0mg
- Sodium: 150mg
- Total Carbohydrates: 12g
- Dietary Fiber: 3g
- Sugars: 2g (includes 0g added sugars)
- Protein: 6g

Cooking Tip: *For a more intense flavor, you can lightly toast the sesame, chia, and flaxseeds in a dry skillet over medium heat for 2-3 minutes before adding them to the mix. Be careful not to burn them. This trail mix is highly customizable, so feel free to add or substitute ingredients according to your taste preferences.*

Recipe 80 - Raspberry Coconut Bars

Prep Time: 15 mins - Cooking Time: 35 mins - Serves: 12

Ingredients:

For the Base:
1 1/2 cups all-purpose flour
1/2 cup unsweetened shredded coconut
1/2 cup granulated sugar
1/2 cup unsalted butter, melted
1/4 teaspoon salt

For the Raspberry Topping:
2 cups fresh raspberries
1/4 cup granulated sugar
1 tablespoon cornstarch
1/4 cup water
1 teaspoon lemon juice

For the Coconut Topping:
1 cup unsweetened shredded coconut
2 tablespoons granulated sugar
1 egg white
1/2 teaspoon vanilla extract

Instructions:
1. Preheat your oven to 350°F (175°C). Line a 9x9 inch baking pan with parchment paper, leaving some overhang for easy removal.
2. Start with the base: In a bowl, mix together flour, 1/2 cup shredded coconut, 1/2 cup sugar, melted butter, and salt until well combined. Press the mixture evenly into the bottom of the prepared pan.
3. Bake the base for 15 minutes until lightly golden. Remove from the oven and let it cool slightly.
4. For the raspberry topping: In a saucepan, combine raspberries, 1/4 cup sugar, cornstarch, water, and lemon juice. Cook over medium heat, stirring constantly, until the mixture thickens and becomes clear. Once thickened, remove from heat and set aside to cool slightly.
5. For the coconut topping: In a separate bowl, combine 1 cup of shredded coconut, 2 tablespoons of sugar, egg whites, and vanilla extract. Mix until well combined.
6. Spread the raspberry mixture evenly over the baked base. Then, gently spread the coconut mixture on top of the raspberry layer.
7. Return the pan to the oven and bake for an additional 20 minutes or until the coconut is lightly golden.
8. Remove from the oven and allow the bars to cool completely in the pan.
9. Once cooled, use the parchment paper overhang to lift out the bars. Cut into squares and serve.

Nutritional Facts (per serving):
- Calories: 280
- Total Fat: 15g
- Saturated Fat: 11g
- Cholesterol: 20mg
- Sodium: 55mg
- Total Carbohydrates: 35g
- Dietary Fiber: 2g
- Sugars: 20g
- Protein: 3g

Recipe 81 - Garlic and Parmesan Roasted Cauliflower

Prep Time: 10 mins - Cooking Time: 25 mins - Serves: 4

Ingredients:
1 large head of cauliflower, cut into bite-sized florets
3 tablespoons olive oil
4 cloves garlic, minced
1/2 cup grated Parmesan cheese
1/2 teaspoon salt
1/4 teaspoon black pepper
1/4 teaspoon red pepper flakes (optional)
2 tablespoons fresh parsley, chopped (for garnish)

Instructions:
1. Preheat your oven to 400°F (200°C). Line a large baking sheet with parchment paper.
2. In a large bowl, toss the cauliflower florets with olive oil and minced garlic, ensuring each piece is well coated.
3. In a small bowl, mix together the grated Parmesan cheese, salt, black pepper, and red pepper flakes (if using).
4. Sprinkle the Parmesan mixture over the cauliflower, tossing it again to coat it evenly.
5. Spread the cauliflower in a single layer on the prepared baking sheet.
6. Roast in the preheated oven for 20-25 minutes or until the cauliflower is tender and the edges are crispy and golden brown. Turn the florets halfway through the cooking time for even roasting.
7. Remove from the oven and sprinkle with fresh parsley for garnish.
8. Serve immediately as a flavorful and crispy side dish.

Nutritional Facts (per serving):
- Calories: 160
- Total Fat: 11g
- Saturated Fat: 3g
- Cholesterol: 11mg
- Sodium: 450mg
- Total Carbohydrates: 10g
- Dietary Fiber: 3g
- Sugars: 3g
- Protein: 7g

Cooking Tip: For extra crispiness, place the roasted cauliflower under the broiler for 2-3 minutes at the end of cooking. Watch closely to prevent burning. The cauliflower can be prepared ahead of time and reheated in the oven for a quick side dish. For a vegan version, substitute Parmesan cheese with nutritional yeast to mimic the cheesy flavor. This recipe is versatile and allows for the addition of other herbs and spices according to your taste preferences.

Recipe 82 - Herbed Wild Rice Pilaf

Prep Time: 10 mins - Cooking Time: 45 mins - Serves: 6

Ingredients:
1 cup wild rice
2 1/2 cups vegetable broth
1 small onion, finely chopped
2 cloves garlic, minced
1/4 cup carrots, diced
1/4 cup celery, diced
1/4 cup fresh parsley, chopped
2 tablespoons fresh thyme, minced
1 tablespoon fresh rosemary, minced
2 tablespoons olive oil
Salt and pepper, to taste
Optional: 1/4 cup dried cranberries or chopped nuts for texture

Instructions:
1. Rinse the wild rice under cold water until the water runs clear.
2. In a medium saucepan, heat the olive oil over medium heat. Add the chopped onion, garlic, carrots, and celery. Sauté for about 5 minutes or until the vegetables are softened.
3. Stir in the wild rice and cook for another 2 minutes, toasting the rice slightly.
4. Add the vegetable broth to the saucepan. Bring the mixture to a boil.
5. Once boiling, reduce the heat to low, cover, and simmer for about 35-45 minutes, or until the rice is tender and has absorbed most of the liquid.
6. Remove from heat and let it sit, covered, for 5 minutes.
7. Fluff the rice with a fork and then stir in the fresh parsley, thyme, and rosemary. Season with salt and pepper to taste.
8. If desired, add dried cranberries or chopped nuts for added texture and flavor.
9. Serve the herbed wild rice pilaf as a delicious and aromatic side dish.

Nutritional Facts (per serving):
- Calories: 180
- Total Fat: 5g
- Saturated Fat: 0.7g
- Cholesterol: 0mg
- Sodium: 410mg
- Total Carbohydrates: 30g
- Dietary Fiber: 3g
- Sugars: 2g
- Protein: 6g

***Cooking Tip**: The key to a flavorful pilaf is to sauté the rice with the vegetables before adding the broth, as this step enhances the rice's nutty flavor. Wild rice can vary in cooking time depending on the brand, so it's important to check the rice for doneness towards the end of cooking. This dish pairs well with a variety of proteins and can be a base for adding other vegetables or proteins to make it a complete meal. Leftovers can be refrigerated and reheated, making it a convenient option for meal prep.*

Recipe 83 - Zucchini and Corn Fritters

Prep Time: 15 mins - Cooking Time: 20 mins - Serves: 4

Ingredients:
2 medium zucchini, grated
1 cup corn kernels (fresh or frozen and thawed)
2 large eggs
1/2 cup all-purpose flour
1/2 teaspoon baking powder
1/4 cup fresh chives, chopped
1/4 cup fresh parsley, chopped
1/2 teaspoon garlic powder
Salt and pepper, to taste
Olive oil for frying

For the Yogurt Dip:
1 cup plain Greek yogurt
1 tablespoon lemon juice
1 clove garlic, minced
2 tablespoons fresh dill, chopped
Salt and pepper, to taste

Instructions:
1. Place the grated zucchini in a colander and sprinkle with a little salt. Let it sit for 10 minutes, then squeeze out as much liquid as possible.
2. In a large bowl, combine the drained zucchini, corn kernels, eggs, flour, baking powder, chives, parsley, garlic powder, salt, and pepper. Stir until well combined.
3. Heat a few tablespoons of olive oil in a large skillet over medium heat.
4. Scoop about 1/4 cup of the zucchini mixture per fritter into the skillet. Flatten them slightly with a spatula.
5. Cook the fritters for 3-4 minutes on each side or until they are golden brown and crispy. Transfer to a paper towel-lined plate to drain any excess oil.
6. For the yogurt dip: In a small bowl, combine Greek yogurt, lemon juice, minced garlic, dill, salt, and pepper. Mix well.
7. Serve the warm zucchini and corn fritters with the yogurt dip on the side.

Nutritional Facts (per serving):
- Calories: 220
- Total Fat: 8g
- Saturated Fat: 2g
- Cholesterol: 95mg
- Sodium: 120mg
- Total Carbohydrates: 27g
- Dietary Fiber: 3g
- Sugars: 6g
- Protein: 12g

***Cooking Tip:** For extra crispiness, make sure the zucchini is well-drained of moisture before mixing with other ingredients. You can also add a bit of grated Parmesan cheese to the fritter mixture for added flavor. These fritters are versatile and can be served as an appetizer, side dish, or light main course. Leftover fritters can be stored in the refrigerator and reheated in a skillet or oven for a quick and tasty snack.*

Recipe 84 - Maple Glazed Carrots

Prep Time: 10 mins - Cooking Time: 25 mins - Serves: 4

Ingredients:
1 pound carrots, peeled and sliced diagonally
3 tablespoons maple syrup
2 tablespoons olive oil
1 tablespoon butter, melted
1/2 teaspoon salt
1/4 teaspoon ground black pepper
Optional: 1/4 teaspoon cinnamon or a pinch of nutmeg
Fresh parsley or thyme for garnish

Instructions:
1. Preheat your oven to 400°F (200°C). Line a baking sheet with parchment paper.
2. In a large bowl, combine the maple syrup, olive oil, melted butter, salt, and black pepper (add cinnamon or nutmeg if using). Mix well.
3. Add the sliced carrots to the bowl and toss them until they are evenly coated with the maple syrup mixture.
4. Spread the carrots out in a single layer on the prepared baking sheet.
5. Roast in the preheated oven for 20-25 minutes, or until the carrots are tender and the edges are caramelized, turning once halfway through cooking.
6. Remove the carrots from the oven and transfer them to a serving dish.
7. Garnish with fresh parsley or thyme before serving.
8. Serve these maple-glazed carrots as a delicious and elegant side dish that complements any meal.

Nutritional Facts (per serving):
- Calories: 150
- Total Fat: 7g
- Saturated Fat: 1.5g
- Cholesterol: 0mg
- Sodium: 320mg
- Total Carbohydrates: 21g
- Dietary Fiber: 3g
- Sugars: 15g
- Protein: 1g

Cooking Tip: *For an extra touch of flavor, you can add a splash of balsamic vinegar to the glaze mixture. The carrots can be cut into different shapes, such as rounds or sticks, for a varied presentation. If you prefer a more savory version, reduce the maple syrup and add garlic powder or smoked paprika. This dish is not only easy to prepare but also makes a visually appealing addition to your dining table. Leftovers can be stored in the refrigerator and reheated or served cold in a salad.*

Recipe 85 - Grilled Vegetable Platter

Prep Time: 15 mins - Cooking Time: 15 mins - Serves: 4-6

Ingredients:
1 red bell pepper, sliced into strips
1 yellow bell pepper, sliced into strips
1 green bell pepper, sliced into strips
1 medium zucchini, sliced lengthwise
1 medium yellow squash, sliced lengthwise
1 medium eggplant, sliced into rounds
2 tablespoons olive oil
2 cloves garlic, minced
1 teaspoon fresh rosemary, chopped
1 teaspoon fresh thyme, chopped
Salt and pepper, to taste
Optional: cherry tomatoes, mushrooms, red onion slices
Fresh parsley or basil for garnish

Instructions:
1. Preheat your grill to medium-high heat.
2. In a large bowl, combine the olive oil, minced garlic, rosemary, thyme, salt, and pepper.
3. Add the sliced bell peppers, zucchini, yellow squash, eggplant, and any other vegetables you're using to the bowl. Toss well to ensure all the vegetables are coated with the herb oil mixture.
4. Place the vegetables on the grill, being careful not to overcrowd the grill. You may need to do this in batches.
5. Grill the vegetables for about 3-5 minutes on each side or until they are tender and have nice grill marks.
6. Once grilled, transfer the vegetables to a serving platter.
7. Garnish with fresh parsley or basil.
8. Serve the grilled vegetable platter as a healthy and colorful side dish or as a part of a larger meal.

Nutritional Facts (per serving):
- Calories: 100
- Total Fat: 7g
- Saturated Fat: 1g
- Cholesterol: 0mg
- Sodium: 50mg
- Total Carbohydrates: 9g
- Dietary Fiber: 3g
- Sugars: 5g
- Protein: 2g

Cooking Tip: For an additional flavor, you can brush the vegetables with balsamic vinegar or a squeeze of lemon juice after grilling. If you don't have a grill, these vegetables can also be roasted in the oven at 425°F (220°C) for about 20 minutes. Feel free to mix and match vegetables based on your preference or what's in season. This platter is not only a feast for the eyes but also a great way to enjoy a variety of vegetables in one meal. Leftovers are great in sandwiches, wraps, or as a topping for salads and pizzas.

Conclusion: Your Transformative Journey Begins Now

In this book, we've delved into the benefits of fasting. It's a method that can truly enhance your well-being, increase your vitality, and help you achieve lasting weight loss. As a reminder, let's review some of the points we've covered in the previous chapters.

Understanding Intermittent Fasting

Intermittent fasting is not considered a diet but rather an eating pattern that involves alternating between periods of fasting and eating. There are approaches to fasting, like the 16/8 method or alternate day fasting, that provide flexibility and can be adjusted to fit individual lifestyles. Fasting initiates responses within the body, such as autophagy, regulation of insulin levels, and the burning of fat.

Health Benefits of Intermittent Fasting

Intermittent fasting has been shown to improve insulin sensitivity, reduce inflammation, and promote cellular health, leading to a decreased risk of chronic diseases such as diabetes, heart disease, and cancer.

Fasting can boost brain function, enhance mental clarity, and potentially reduce the risk of neurodegenerative diseases.

Intermittent fasting can also support weight loss by promoting fat burning, preserving muscle mass, and regulating appetite hormones.

Implementing Intermittent Fasting

To successfully adopt fasting, it is important to make changes. Begin by extending your fasting period and then slowly increase the duration of your fasting window. It is crucial to stay hydrated during your fasting periods. Remember to consume a certain amount of water, herbal teas, or other non-caloric beverages. It's also important to pay attention to your body's signals and make adjustments to your fasting schedule as necessary. Finding a rhythm that suits your needs is essential.

Encouragement to start the intermittent fasting journey.

Now that you've developed an understanding of fasting and its many benefits, it's time to take the plunge and begin your transformative journey. Starting fasting may feel overwhelming at first. Armed with the knowledge and tools presented in this book, you're fully equipped to embrace this lifestyle change. Remember, the path towards a happier version of yourself starts with that step.

As you embark on your fasting journey, keep these words of encouragement in mind:

Embrace the Process: Transformations don't happen overnight. Intermittent fasting isn't a fix; it's a shift in lifestyle. Embrace the process, practice patience, and trust in your journey. Celebrate every victory along the way.

Practice Self-Compassion: Be kind to yourself throughout this process. There may be days where slip-ups occur or sticking to your fasting schedule becomes challenging. Remember that it's about progress rather than perfection. Treat each day as an opportunity for renewed focus and commitment.

Seek Support and Accountability: Sharing your fasting experience with others can be incredibly empowering. Look for support from friends, family members, or online communities who can offer guidance, accountability, and motivation. Together, you can celebrate achievements. Tackle any obstacles that come your way.

Be attentive and attuned to your body: Intermittent fasting doesn't have a formula that works for everyone. It's important to listen to your body's cues and adapt your fasting routine accordingly. Stay aware of your hunger, energy levels, and overall well-being. Remember, taking care of yourself is a part of this transformative process.

Final thoughts and empowering message for readers.

As we come to the end of this book, I'd like to share a message of empowerment. You hold the ability to make changes in your health, body, and life. Intermittent fasting goes beyond being a tool; it's a pathway that unlocks your potential. By adopting this lifestyle change, you are actively prioritizing your well-being. Taking charge of your destiny.

Remember that your journey is unique, and there's is no need to compare yourself to others. Focus on your progress. Celebrate every milestone you reach. Trust in the power of fasting and its remarkable impact on your physical, mental, and emotional well-being.

The road ahead may have its ups and downs. Always keep in mind why you embarked on this journey in the place. Tap into your strength, resilience, and determination to overcome any obstacles that may arise along the way. You possess the strength to achieve your goals, with fasting as a guiding force for initiating this transformative journey.

So take that step forward, embrace the power of intermittent fasting wholeheartedly, and witness your health, energy levels, and overall vitality soar higher than ever before. You are capable; you are resilient; you are prepared. Your incredible journey awaits.

Appendix: Frequently Asked Questions about Intermittent Fasting

In this section, we will tackle frequently asked questions about fasting, giving you an understanding of this eating approach and its potential advantages. We will also provide sources. Suggested readings for further exploration, along with a glossary of terms to improve your knowledge of intermittent fasting.

Frequently Asked Questions

Q: What is intermittent fasting?

A: Intermittent fasting refers to an eating pattern that involves alternating between periods of fasting and eating. It's not about what you eat. When you eat. There are methods, such as the 16/8 method (fasting for 16 hours and restricting eating to an 8-hour window) and the 5:2 method (eating normally for five days and limiting calorie intake to 500 to 600 calories on two non-consecutive days).

Q: Does fasting work effectively for weight loss?

A: Yes, intermittent fasting has proven to be effective for weight loss. Narrowing down the eating window or reducing calorie intake on days can create a calorie deficit, which leads to weight loss. Additionally, intermittent fasting may enhance metabolism, improve insulin sensitivity, and promote burning.

Q: Can I still build muscle while practicing fasting?

A: Absolutely! It is indeed possible to build muscle while following a fasting routine. Ensuring adequate protein intake along with resistance training can help preserve existing muscle mass and even facilitate its growth. However, it's crucial to prioritize nutrition during the designated eating window in order to support muscle development.

Q: Is fasting for everyone?

A: Although intermittent fasting can offer advantages to people, it may not be suitable for everyone.. Breastfeeding women, individuals with medical conditions, and those who have a history of disordered eating should be cautious or seek guidance from a healthcare professional before adopting this eating pattern.

Q: What are the health benefits of fasting?

A: Intermittent fasting has demonstrated benefits beyond weight loss. These include improved insulin sensitivity, reduced inflammation, enhanced brain function, increased cellular repair and regeneration (known as autophagy), and increased longevity. Some research even suggests that it may lower the risk of diseases like type 2 diabetes and heart disease.

Additional Resources and Recommended Readings

"The Obesity Code" by Dr. Jason Fung - A comprehensive guide exploring the factors contributing to obesity and how intermittent fasting can help.

"Delay, Don't Deny" by Gin Stephens - Offers personal insights and practical tips for successful intermittent fasting.

"The Complete Guide to Fasting" by Dr. Jason Fung and Jimmy Moore - An in-depth resource discussing various fasting methods and their potential health benefits.

"Intermittent Fasting for Beginners" by Amanda Swaine is a beginner-friendly guide to understanding and implementing intermittent fasting in your lifestyle.

Glossary of Definitions

Autophagy: It's a process where the body breaks down damaged cells and recycles them, which helps maintain health and longevity.

Insulin Sensitivity: This refers to the body's ability to effectively respond to insulin, which helps regulate blood sugar levels and lowers the risk of insulin resistance and type 2 diabetes.

Calorie Deficit: It means consuming more calories than our body needs, resulting in weight loss.

Eating Window: This refers to the period during which one consumes food and drinks while practicing fasting.

In this appendix, we've addressed some questions about fasting. We've also included resources for those who want to explore the topic and a glossary of important terms related to this eating pattern. Intermittent fasting has become popular because of its advantages for weight loss, metabolism, and overall well-being. It's essential to consult with a healthcare expert before adopting any dietary or fasting routine to make sure it suits your needs and goals.

About The Author

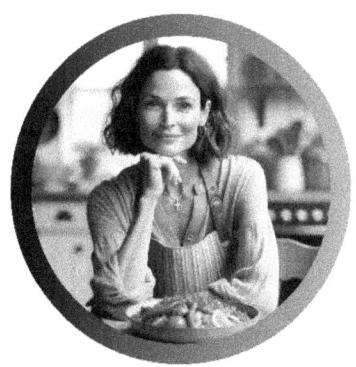

Samantha Bax, an advocate of vegan, eco-mindful cuisine, discovered her true passion in the heart of a bustling city. However, her culinary journey didn't start in a kitchen but rather in her grandmother's cozy home, where she first learned the importance of nourishing and wholesome eating.

When Samantha was diagnosed with diabetes during her twenties, her life took a turn. This pivotal moment fueled her commitment to health and well-being, leading her to become a certified nutritionist. Fate had something in store for Samantha when a close family member was diagnosed with kidney disease. This significant event brought together her two passions. Food and wellness. Inspiring her to create a niche that caters to both renal diets.

Course Samantha faced challenges along the way. Balancing health requirements while maintaining flavors proved to be quite complex. However, she remained steadfast in refusing to compromise taste for the sake of health. To overcome this obstacle, Samantha embarked on an adventure where she sought inspiration from kitchens across the Mediterranean region, vibrant spice markets in Asia, and sustainable farms throughout Central America.

In *"Intermittent Fasting For Women Over 50,"* Samantha Bax beautifully intertwines her story with an enticing collection of mouth-watering recipes.

She strongly believes that food is not a means of survival. Also, it is something to be cherished as a way to celebrate life and promote well-being.

The main aim of her book is to present readers with a curated collection of recipes that cater to their needs while also providing them with an enjoyable culinary experience.

Apart from writing and experimenting in the kitchen, Samantha finds joy in the art of photography. She skillfully captures the essence of cityscapes, as well as serene landscapes, in nature. Furthermore, she actively leads workshops and seminars where she guides individuals on how to make food choices that prioritize taste without compromising on quality.

To join our Newsletter and receive advance notification of new publications, subscribe to the Newsletter for FREE today at:

www.prosebooks.us/subscribe

Other Books by Samantha Bax

No. 23-1065   1200-Calorie Diet For Senior Women: Lose Weight, Improve Your Health, And Live Longer With a 1200-Calorie Meal Plan Daily

No. 23-1082   Celiac Disease Cookbook For The Newly Diagnosed: Guide To Cooking Easy And Delicious Gluten-Free Recipes For Everyone With Celiac Disease

No. 23-1078   Fasting Your Way to Better Blood Sugar: The Ultimate Blueprint For Effortless Weight Management And Insulin Resistance With Intermittent Fasting And Zero Sugar Diet For Diabetes Patients

No. 23-1076   Fatty Liver Diet Cookbook For Seniors Over 50: Fatty Liver Diet Cookbook For Seniors Over 50

No 23-1079   Intermittent Fasting For Seniors: A Beginner's Guide To Losing 10 to 30 Pounds For Senior Men And Women In 3 months. Healthy Recipes Tailored With All Diets During Your Fasting

No. 23-1075   Intermittent Fasting For Women With PCOS: The Science-Based Guide for Using Intermittent Fasting to Conquer PCOS, diabetes, prediabetes, Lose Weight, Balance Hormones, Increase Energy, and more

No. 23-1071   Low Histamine Diet Cookbook And Meal Plan: Hope and Healing In Your Kitchen: Gluten-Free and Anti-Inflammatory Recipes For Histamine Intolerance

No. 23-1070   Ninja Speedi Keto Cookbook: Lightning Quick Keto Meals for Busy Lives - Make the Most of Your Ninja Speedi with These Fuss-Free Keto Recipes

No. 23-1069   Ninja Speedi Keto Cookbook: From Fridge to Table in a Flash - 150+ Quick and Delicious Recipes for Your Ninja Speedi

No. 23-1074   Osteoporosis Diet Cookbook For Men: The Complete Guide to Preventing and Reversing Bone Loss with Delicious and Nutritious Recipes

No. 23-1073   Osteoporosis Diet Cookbook Recipes For Seniors: Delicious and Nutritious Science-Based and Calcium Fortified Recipes for Men and Women with Osteoporosis

No. 23-1080   Plant-Based Kidney Disease Diet Cookbook For Beginners: Beginner Friendly Low-Sodium Recipes And Guides To Prevent And Manage Chronic Kidney Disease (CKD) And Avoid Dialysis

No. 23-1081   Pritikin Diet For Seniors: The Complete Guide To Weight Loss And Improved Health For Seniors

No. 23-1066   Vegan Diabetic Renal Diet Cookbook: 125+ Delicious And Nutritious Low Sodium And Low Potassium Recipes To Help You Manage Your Diabetes And Cure Kidney Disease

No. 23-1077   Vegan Diabetic Renal Diet Cookbook (2nd Edition): 125+ Delicious And Nutritious Low Sodium And Low Potassium Recipes To Help You Manage Your Diabetes And Cure Kidney Disease

See all of Samantha Bax's books here: https://prosebooks.us/books

Scan the above code to see all the books and more…

https://prosebooks.us/books

Thank You

Dear Reader,

As we approach the end of this journey, I want to express my sincere gratitude to you for embracing these recipes in your kitchen and, in turn, in your life. Your support means the world to me. It ignites my passion for sharing the goodness that food brings to our tables and our souls.

May the flavors you've explored and the nourishment you've derived from these pages inspire moments of happiness, connection, and well-being. Always remember that every meal you prepare is an expression of your imagination and thoughtfulness.

Looking forward to our escapade,

Warmest regards,

Samantha Bax

BONUS: FREE Meal-Planner

As a FREE Bonus to all my readers, I invite you to go to my publisher's website at www.prosebooks.us/meal-planner and get a FREE Meal Planner to help and guide you along your journey to fitness and good health.

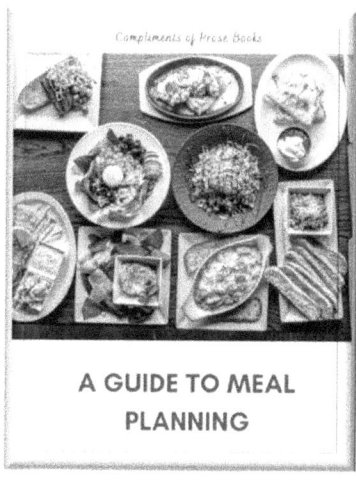

www.ingramcontent.com/pod-product-compliance
Lightning Source LLC
Chambersburg PA
CBHW081253040426
42453CB00014B/2394